Gulsheen Kaur Kochhar
Inder Kumar Pandit
Amandeep Singh Uppal

Caries Removal Techniques in Primary Teeth

Gulsheen Kaur Kochhar
Inder Kumar Pandit
Amandeep Singh Uppal

Caries Removal Techniques in Primary Teeth

A Comparitive Clinical Evaluation of Different Caries Removal Techniques in Primary Teeth

LAP LAMBERT Academic Publishing

Impressum / Imprint

Bibliografische Information der Deutschen Nationalbibliothek: Die Deutsche Nationalbibliothek verzeichnet diese Publikation in der Deutschen Nationalbibliografie; detaillierte bibliografische Daten sind im Internet über http://dnb.d-nb.de abrufbar.

Alle in diesem Buch genannten Marken und Produktnamen unterliegen warenzeichen-, marken- oder patentrechtlichem Schutz bzw. sind Warenzeichen oder eingetragene Warenzeichen der jeweiligen Inhaber. Die Wiedergabe von Marken, Produktnamen, Gebrauchsnamen, Handelsnamen, Warenbezeichnungen u.s.w. in diesem Werk berechtigt auch ohne besondere Kennzeichnung nicht zu der Annahme, dass solche Namen im Sinne der Warenzeichen- und Markenschutzgesetzgebung als frei zu betrachten wären und daher von jedermann benutzt werden dürften.

Bibliographic information published by the Deutsche Nationalbibliothek: The Deutsche Nationalbibliothek lists this publication in the Deutsche Nationalbibliografie; detailed bibliographic data are available in the Internet at http://dnb.d-nb.de.

Any brand names and product names mentioned in this book are subject to trademark, brand or patent protection and are trademarks or registered trademarks of their respective holders. The use of brand names, product names, common names, trade names, product descriptions etc. even without a particular marking in this works is in no way to be construed to mean that such names may be regarded as unrestricted in respect of trademark and brand protection legislation and could thus be used by anyone.

Coverbild / Cover image: www.ingimage.com

Verlag / Publisher:
LAP LAMBERT Academic Publishing
ist ein Imprint der / is a trademark of
AV Akademikerverlag GmbH & Co. KG
Heinrich-Böcking-Str. 6-8, 66121 Saarbrücken, Deutschland / Germany
Email: info@lap-publishing.com

Herstellung: siehe letzte Seite /
Printed at: see last page
ISBN: 978-3-659-24329-5

Copyright © 2012 AV Akademikerverlag GmbH & Co. KG
Alle Rechte vorbehalten. / All rights reserved. Saarbrücken 2012

CONTENTS

1. Introduction..................................Page 3
2. Review of Literature..........................Page 7
3. Materials and Methods........................Page 17
4. Observations and Results....................Page 34
5. Discussion...................................Page 51
6. Conclusion..................................Page 73
7. References..................................Page 74
9. Appendix....................................Page 84

INTRODUCTION

The word "caries" is derived from the Latin word meaning "rot" and Greek word "ker" meaning death.[1] According to WHO, caries is defined as "localized post erupted, pathological process of external origin involving softening of hard tooth tissue and proceeding to the formation of a cavity."[2]

Dental Caries has affected mankind since pre-historic times and is still one of the most common diseases of modern civilization. It is a biosocial disease, known to affect the patients of all age groups, religions, regions, socio-economic status & both the sexes. Both primary and permanent teeth can be affected by the wrath of dental caries and according to the recent oral health survey in India; 50-55% of the population is affected from caries, with an average DMFT of 2.7-3.1. The prevalence is higher in urban areas than in rural and more in girls than in boys.[3]

Various efforts for prevention of dental caries are being undertaken at global levels but still it continues to affect a significant portion of the world population. It is asymptomatic in initial stages but may cause discomfort and pain as it progresses. When caries is confined to enamel, various conservative approaches like enameloplasty, atraumatic restorative treatment etc. can be done. However, once caries progresses to deeper layers of enamel or dentin, the only option left is to excavate the carious tooth structure and to restore it with appropriate restorative material.

The most primitive method of caries excavation has been by using hand instruments. The early hand instruments, with their large heavy handles and inferior metal alloys on the blades, were cumbersome and ineffective in many situations. More so, excavation by hand instruments is painful, ineffective and tedious procedure.

To overcome these drawbacks, modern rotary instruments were developed with the manufacturing of powered foot engine. Due to heavy weight of the drill and low speed, electric motors were introduced. Initially, removal of carious dentin was performed mechanically with the burs in low speed hand pieces (<12000rpm) but in recent years, high speed rotary equipments having approximately 300,000rpm are being used.[4] Exclusive use of high-speed excavation with air turbine hand pieces removes both infected and non-infected dentin, which may cause an excessive cutting and unnecessary weakness of the tooth structure, and may also increase the possibilities of damaging pulpal tissue. These invasive methods of treating dental caries despite of being quick and efficient resulted in pain and discomfort due to heat, vibration and noise. In addition, these cause deleterious thermal and pressure effects on the pulp and contribute to pain and anxiety especially in children.[5]

Till recent past, silver amalgam was the material of choice for restoration. Cavity preparation for silver amalgam was based on Dr. G.V. Black's principle of "Extension for Prevention". However, due to shortcomings of drill and overcutting of tooth structure associated with silver amalgam restorations, there has been a growing interest in the development of alternative techniques which apart from being more comfortable preserve healthy dental tissues.[6]

Lately, with the introduction of new adhesive restorative materials, various minimal invasive techniques have been developed with the aim of elimination of carious lesions and maximum preservation of healthy tooth structure. These include air abrasion, sonoabrasion, ultrasonic instrumentation, lasers and chemomechanical approach of caries removal. Of these air abrasions, sonoabrasion, ultrasonic instrumentation, lasers are not cost effective and therefore, are less frequently used.[7]

Chemo-mechanical approach is an alternative to traditional drilling. It minimizes sound tissue removal as it is more selective, self limiting and prevents permanent damage of dentin layers by avoiding heating and vibration produced by rotary instruments and making it less painful.[7]

The procedure involves the application of chemical solution to the carious dentin followed by gentle removal with hand instruments. It is comfortable for the patients, easy to use, noiseless and painless. **Fernanda NPC et al 2007** stated that the objective of chemo mechanical substances was to remove the most external portion (infected layer) of carious tooth structure, leaving behind the affected demineralized dentin that was capable of remineralisation and repair.[8]

Chemo-mechanical caries removal system involves the use of substances like Carisolv and Papacarie. Carisolv is marketed as a gel and consists of 3 amino acids-lysine, leucine and glutamic acid along with a solution of sodium hypochlorite. It removes caries by selectively reacting with the denatured collagen thereby making carious dentin soft without affecting healthy dentin.[9]

Recently, in 2003, Papacarie a material composed of papain, chloramine and toluidine blue was launched to be used as chemomechanical caries removal method. Papain is an endoprotein with bacteriostatic, bactericidal and anti-inflammatory activity. Chloramine, contains chlorine and ammonia, possessing bactericidal and disinfectant properties which is used to irrigate root canals and to chemically soften carious dentin. The degraded portion of carious dentin collagen is chlorinated by the solution, which helps in chemical and mechanical caries removal.[10]

Despite the availability of various methods and materials for caries removal, the most preferable method of caries removal in pediatric patients would be the one which is painless and which effectively removes soft carious tooth structure without unnecessary pain.

Regardless of the fact that the newer chemomechanical methods of caries removal are comfortable and acceptable, there is still lack of adequate clinical studies comparing the efficacy and adequacy with conventional methods for caries removal in pediatric patients. Therefore, the present study was undertaken to compare the clinical efficacy of chemomechanical caries removal with conventional caries removal methods in children.

REVIEW OF LITERATURE

Dental caries has been and still continues to be among the most commonly occurring dental diseases in the world. There are a number of techniques available for the removal of caries. Most primitive approach to the treatment of caries was by hand instruments which was a painful, ineffective and tedious method. This later on led to the evolution of rotary instruments initially, from low speed to ultra high speed. During their use the thermal and pressure effects on the pulp produced pain, a major drawback with this technique. Therefore, there has been a growing interest in developing alternative techniques for caries removal e.g. chemomechanical techniques, lasers etc.

The following review highlights the studies conducted on the various caries removal methods:

ATRAUMATIC RESTORATIVE TECHNIQUES:

- ➢ The extent of discomfort with atraumatic restorative treatment of multisurface cavities in primary molars was compared with that of rotary instruments by **Schriks MCM et al (2003)**[11]. Results confirmed that children treated according to the ART approach using hand instruments alone experienced less discomfort than those treated with rotary instruments.

- ➢ **Lopez N et al 2004**[12] evaluated the acceptability and effectiveness of atraumatic restorative treatment to prevent and treat caries in an underserved community in Mexico. After 2-year evaluation, 66% of restorations and 35% of sealants were retained and it was concluded that atraumatic restorative treatment was acceptable and effective to control and prevent decay in a socioeconomically deprived community.

- **Frencken JE et al 2004**[13] used a minimal intervention approach to manage dental caries. They concluded that Atraumatic Restorative Treatment (ART) appeared to be less painful and more patient friendly than conventional caries treatment. It was also effective for the management of single surface cavities in both primary and permanent dentitions. They also concluded that ART approach was beneficial in improving the oral health of many, not only in developing but also in more advanced countries

- **Deery C et al 2005**[14] conducted a survey in children with at least one multisurface cavity in a primary molar. The test group was treated using atraumatic restorative techniques (ART) using only hand instruments and the control group received treatment using rotary instruments (operated at 750 rpm), without water cooling. Glass ionomer cement was used for restoration in both the groups. Children treated according to the ART approach using hand instruments experienced less discomfort than those treated using rotary instruments.

- **Ersin et al 2006**[15] conducted a study to examine the changes in the cultivable microflora of carious dentin before and after atraumatic restorative treatment (ART) and investigate the inhibitory effect of chlorhexidine-gluconate-based cavity disinfectant in the microflora. It was concluded that ART was effective in reducing the cultivable microflora and also it was found that chlorhexidine-gluconate-based cavity disinfectant might serve as a suitable additional agent in inhibiting the residual bacteria in the dentin.

- Study conducted by **Toi CS et al 2009**[16] determined the effectiveness of ART in removing carious tissue, by investigating the numbers of mutans Streptococci and lactobacilli, with emphasis on the prevalence of

Streptococcus mutans and Streptococcus sobrinus strains before and after ART treatment of dental caries. The significant decrease in bacteria after manual cavity preparation demonstrated the reliability of a standardized ART technique. But the presence of S.mutans strains showed that the effectiveness of the ART procedure could vary during treatment and between dental practitioners.

- **Mickenautsch S et al 2009**[17] conducted a study to report the longevity of restorations placed using the atraumatic restorative treatment (ART) approach compared with that of amalgam restorations. Results showed that restorations placed in the primary dentition showed no significant differences between the groups after 12 and 24 months. In the permanent dentition, the longevity of ART restorations was equal to or greater than that of equivalent amalgam restorations for up to 6.3 years and was site dependent whereas no difference was observed in primary teeth.

ROTARY MECHANICAL METHOD

- **Walkens CE (1965)**[18] investigated the effectiveness of an air coolant in ultra high speed cutting of tooth structure. Maintenance of the intra-pulpal temperature as close to 0 as possible was of great importance during grinding procedures, in which ultra high speeds were used. The problem of access and vision dictated the use of a flexible cooling armamentarium, enhancing the procedure.

- **Lester KS et al 1978**[19] substantiated that scanning electron microscope studies demonstrated deficiencies in the surfaces of cavity preparations made with conventional cutting instruments. Better surface preparation was achieved by using appropriate shaped tungsten rotary instruments, and by sharp hand instruments used with scraping action. The direction of rotation of cutting alters the quality of enamel margin.

- **Boston DW (2003)[20]** conducted a study to develop prototype rotary selective dentin caries excavators and to demonstrate their ability to remove only carious dentin in extracted teeth. Milled polymer prototype and formed wire loop prototype burs were made. They were tested on normal dentin with standardized force application and were compared to carbide burs for their ability to cut. Both the prototypes removed carious dentin but did not remove normal dentin in the extracted teeth.

- **Antunes AAA et al 2008[21]** conducted a study to compare the effectiveness of high speed (HS) and air abrasion (AA) instruments on groups of teeth, in terms of preparation time, topography and presence of smear layer. In conclusion, the High Speed instrument was found to be more rapid than the Air Abrasion. No difference was found with respect to the topography and the presence of smear layer. The differences found in the present study were only in relation to the effects of each instrument used.

CHEMO-MECHANICAL CARIES REMOVAL: CARISOLV

- **Goldman M et al (1975)[22]** did a comparative in-vitro study of GK 101 (N-monochloroglycine) and GK 101 E (ethyl derivative of GK 101), in caries removal, on extracted carious human teeth. This study indicated that both GK 101 and GK 101 E exerted a statistically significant chemical action in the removal of the caries material. GK 101 was statistically superior to saline in caries removal in medium-hard lesions. It was not statistically superior to saline in lesions of medium consistency.

> **Ericsona D et al 1999**[23] clinically evaluated the efficacy and safety of newer methods of chemomechanical removal of caries, Carisolv and concluded that dentin caries was effectively removed using the Carisolv method without any adverse reactions.

> **Beeley JA et al 2000**[7] stated chemomechanical caries removal involved the chemical softening of carious dentin followed by its removal by gentle excavation. The reagent involved was generated by mixing amino acids with sodium hypochlorite; N-monochloroamino acids was formed which selectively degraded demineralized collagen in carious dentin. The procedure required 5-15 minutes but avoided the painful removal of sound dentin thereby reducing the need for local anesthesia. It was well suited for the treatment of primary teeth, dental phobics and medically compromised patients. The dentin surface formed was highly irregular and well suited for bonding with composite resin or glass ionomer. When complete caries removal was achieved, the dentin remaining was sound and properly mineralized. The system was originally marketed in USA in the 1980's as Caridex. Large volumes of solution and a special applicator system were required. A new system, Carisolv, was launched in to the market which comes as a gel that required volumes of 0.2–1.0 ml and was also accompanied by specially designed instruments.

> **Maragakis GM et al 2001**[24] evaluated the clinical efficiency and patient acceptance of the chemomechanical caries removal agent Carisolv^{TM} in primary teeth. It was concluded that, Carisolv, although a step forward in terms of solution volume required, was not in a position to replace rotary instruments for caries removal. It did not remove decay completely in one third of our samples, it was much slower than the Airotor and it had a chlorine taste/odor our patients disliked.

- A study was conducted to determine the clinical evaluation of Carisolv in chemo-mechanical removal of carious dentin by **Munshi AK et al (2001)**[9]. They demonstrated that Carisolv is effective atraumatic treatment modality for the use in pediatric dentistry.
- **Burrow MF et al 2002**[25] compared the microtensile bond strengths of two resin-based adhesives, conventional glass ionomer cement and resin modified glass ionomer cement to normal and caries affected dentin after Carisolv treatment. It was concluded that carious dentin treated with Carisolv did not affect the adhesion of the adhesive restorative materials tested in this study with the exception of Fuji II LC.
- **Sakoolnamarka R et al 2002**[26] conducted morphological study of demineralized dentin after caries removal using two different methods. Six teeth had caries removed using burs after staining with a caries detector dye, and caries from the others was removed using Carisolv. From this study it was shown that etched normal dentin and etched caries-affected dentin had different surface appearances. Furthermore, the two caries removal techniques resulted in different caries-affected dentin surfaces after acid treatment that influenced the longevity of bonds from adhesive restorative materials.
- **Rafique et al 2003**[27] conducted a study to investigate whether caries removal with air-abrasion/ Carisolv™ gel was an acceptable and viable alternative in the treatment of dental patients. Results showed that Carisolv gel was an acceptable alternative method of caries removal in terms of time taken, pain/discomfort and taste. The conclusion drawn from the study was that air-abrasion/Carisolv gel treatment was a well-accepted and viable

alternative to conventional local anesthetic injection and drill for dental patients.

- In vitro comparison of the efficacy of Carisolv™ and conventional rotary instrument in caries removal was done by **Yazici AR et al 2003**[28]. The purpose of this in vitro study was to compare the efficacy of a new chemomechanical caries removal agent, Carisolv™ (MediTeam AB, Savedalen, Sweden), with conventional slow-speed rotary instrument (bur). The results of this study suggest that conventional rotary instrument (bur) was more effective than Carisolv in removal of carious tissue and also takes shorter time.

- **Azark B et al (2004)**[29] conducted a study to compare the efficacy of chemomechanical caries removal (Carisolv) with that of conventional excavation in reducing the cariogenic flora and their results indicated that efficacy of chemomechanical removal of carious dentin in children by means of Carisolv was comparable to results obtained by conventional methods and thus, might serve as a suitable alternative.

- **Fluckiger L et al 2004**[30] conducted a study to compare the efficacy of chemomechanical caries removal (Carisolv) and conventional hand excavation in primary teeth. It was concluded that the Carisolv method was significantly more time consuming than conventional preparation using hand excavator. However, both methods removed caries efficiently.

- **Balciuniene I et al 2005**[31] conducted a study to evaluate the new chemomechanical method of caries removal using Carisolv® gel for primary and permanent teeth of children comparing it with traditional caries removing by rotary instruments and to determine the need of anesthetics. It was concluded that using Carisolv® gel the number of complaints of pain declined more than twice, which meant that this method was much less painful than traditional method of drilling. The chemomechanical method had no problems of unpleasant taste or unpleasant smell and the average mean of cleaning time was longer than in traditional treatment group.

- **Peters MC et al (2006)[32]** investigated the effectiveness of chemomechanical caries removal (CMCR) compared with the traditional methods(TM) of caries removal using a round bur when treating dentinal-depth occlusal lesions with minimal enamel access in primary molars. It concluded that there was no direct advantage of using CMCR over using TM for treating occlusal dentinal lesions with minimal cavitations in pediatric patients.

- **Chourio MAL et al 2006[33]** conducted a study to compare the chemomechanical caries-removal system (Carisolv™) with high-speed excavation in cavitated occlusal caries of primary molars. Results showed that time taken for caries removal was three times longer. Some pain was reported by participants when Carisolv was used but it was less when compared with high-speed excavation. Using the Carisolv method there was a higher proportion of patients with positive behavior. It was concluded that Carisolv was an effective clinical alternative treatment for the removal of occlusal dentinal caries in cavitated primary molars; it was more conservative for dental tissue and appeared to be more comfortable for most patients, although the clinical time spent was longer than when using high-speed excavation.

- **Pandit IK et al 2007[34]** compared the different methods of caries removal in children of age group 6-9 years. Caries removal was done by Hand instruments, Airotor and Carisolv. The efficacy, time taken and pain experienced by the patient during caries removal was evaluated. Results showed that Airotor was the most efficient method (mean value 0.38), while

Carisolv was the least painful (mean value 0.080) and the most time consuming method (534.8 seconds).

- Study conducted by **Inglehart MR et al 2007**[35] investigated operators and pediatric patients responses to chemo-mechanical caries removal (CMCR) versus the traditional method (TM) of caries removal using a handpiece and a round bur when treating dentinal depth occlusal lesions with minimal enamel access in primary molars. It was concluded that using CMCR required more clinical and technical effort and more overall effort than using TM. Therefore operator's satisfaction with using CMCR was lower than with using TM.

- **Subramaniam P et al 2008**[36] evaluated the antimicrobial efficacy of chemomechanical caries removal (Carisolv™) in reducing the count of cariogenic flora and compared it to conventional drilling. Results indicated that the antimicrobial efficacy of Carisolv™ was comparable to that of conventional drilling and could be used as a suitable alternative for caries removal, especially in children.

CHEMO-MECHANICAL CARIES REMOVAL: PAPACARIE

- **Bussadori SK et al (2005)**[10] stated that the chemo-mechanical caries removal method has been a solution for patient seeking alternatives to conventional methods. Among different kinds of chemo-mechanical caries removal systems, Papacarie-a papain gel was found to be easy to manipulate, simple and cheap, as well as effective in removing infected tissues.

- Another in vitro study conducted by **Correa FN et al (2007)**[8] assessed the remaining dentinal surface after carious tooth tissue removal with a low speed conventional bur and two chemomechanical methods, (PapacárieTM and Carisolv®), using the microhardness test. It was concluded that the hardness of the remaining dentin after carious tissue removal was lower than that obtained on healthy dentin, without significant difference between the various means of carious tissue removal.

- **Carrillo CM et al 2008**[37] evaluated complete caries removal time (CCR) and patient acceptance of the chemomechanical caries removal agent and papain gel Papacarie in disabled patients and results emphasized that Papacarie gel had complete caries removal time of 8 minutes per tooth and was well accepted by the patients in all phases and in the first and subsequent visits.
- **Bussadori K et al 2008**[38] presented a paper proposing the use of a papain-based gel for the removal of active caries with infected tissue followed by a glass ionomer restoration in an adolescent patient. Removal of caries tissue with Papacarie® proved to be efficient, easy and comfortable for the patient.
- **Motta LJ et al 2009**[39] presented a clinical case of aesthetic restoration of both upper primary central incisors after the removal of carious tissue with Papacárie®. Chemomechanical caries removal was a conservative and atraumatic alternative. Papacárie®, a papain-based material developed to act only on the carious dentin, allowing its easy removal with a blunt curette. It was concluded that the use of Papacárie® for the removal of carious tissue represents an alternative for dental cavity preparation. It promoted better preservation of healthy tissue and reduced the disadvantages of conventional methods using dental drills and excavators that induced discomfort and pain. It's an appropriate procedure in pediatric dentistry.

MATERIALS AND METHODS

The present study was conducted in department of Pedodontics and Preventive Dentistry, D.A.V (C) Dental College & Hospital, Yamuna Nagar. This in vivo study was conducted to evaluate and compare the efficacy of different methods of caries removal that is Hand instruments, Airotor, Carisolv gel and Papacarie gel in children.

MATERIALS (Fig.1)

(A) CARISOLV GEL

Carisolv gel Uncolored Multimix (Mediteam Dental AB, Sweden). It consists of a twin syringe, with an end cap, plunger and static mixer for dispensing the gel.

Composition:

Syringe 1-

The gel comprises uncolored fluid of high viscosity, which contains three different amino acids; glutamic acid, leucine, lysine.

- Carboxymethylcellulose that enhances the viscosity.
- Sodium hydroxide, which provides a pH of 11.
- Sodium chloride and purified water as a vehicle.

Syringe 2 –

A transparent fluid, which consists of 0.95% sodium hypochlorite

(B) PAPACARIE GEL

Papacarie (F& A Laboratorio Farmaceutico Ltd.) available as 3ml solution.

Composition:

- Papain
- Chloramines
- Toluidine blue
- Salts
- Preservatives
- Vehicle qsp.

(C) OTHER MATERIALS

1. Caries detecting dye – Caries detector

    (Kuraray Medical Inc., Tokyo, Japan)

    Composition:

    1% acid red in propylene glycol

2. Glass Ionomer Cement (GC-Fuji II)

    Composition: Powder : Fluoro-alumino silicate glass – 95%,

    Polyacrylic acid powder -5%

    Liquid : Distilled water – 50%

    Polyacrylic acid – 40 %

    Polybasic carboxylic acid

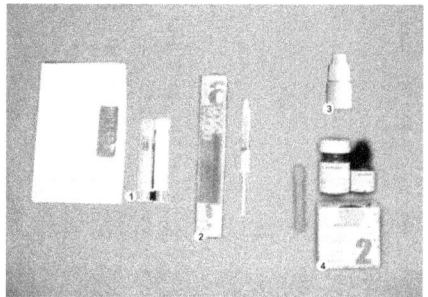

Fig.1: Materials :1.Carisolv gel, 2. Papacarie gel, 3. Caries detecting dye, 4.Glass Ionomer Cement

ARMAMENTARIUM (Fig.2)

The following armamentarium was used for various methods of caries removal

(A) FOR HAND INSTRUMENTS:

Spoon excavator (Hu-friedy, USA)

(B) FOR AIROTOR:

1. Contra-angled high-speed air rotor hand-piece, with water as coolant (NSK. PANA AIR-Σ).
2. Diamond cutting burs (d=1mm) - round bur (ADA no.2), straight fissure, inverted cone (ADA no.33.5).

(C) FOR CARIES REMOVAL BY CARISOLV:

Hand instruments with interchangeable tips (Mediteam, Sweden) were used for gel application and removal of caries.

(D) FOR CARIES REMOVAL BY PAPACARIE:

Spoon excavator (API)

(E) MISCELLANEOUS ARMAMENTARIUM:

1. X-ray Grid
2. Mouth mirror (API)
3. DG-16 Probe (Hu-friedy, USA)
4. Explorer (API 99/578)
5. Tweezer (API 99/519)
6. Cotton
7. Plastic filling instrument
8. Suction tip
9. Rubber and kit (Hygienic, Dental Dam Kit-Fiesta 9Color Wingless)
10. Agate Spatula, Mixing pad, Mylar strip
11. Articulating paper (Samit products)
12. Composite finishing burs (Shofu Inc.,Japan)
13. Stop Watch

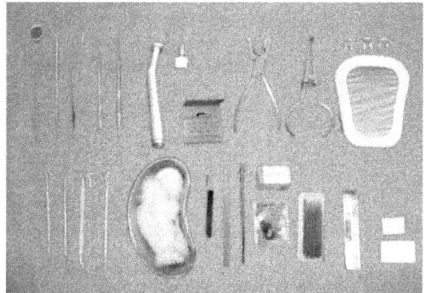

Fig.2: Armamentarium.

METHODOLOGY

SELECTION OF THE PATIENTS

A total number of 80 patients in the age group of 5-9 years were selected from the Out Patient Department of Pedodontics, Preventive and Community Dentistry, D.A.V (C) Dental College and Hospital, Yamuna Nagar, who on intraoral examination were found to have single or multiple carious primary teeth on either surface were selected. Only the teeth with single carious lesion were considered. Before selection, all teeth were judged according to the following inclusion and exclusion criteria. Only the patients who fulfilled the following inclusion and exclusion criteria were selected for the study.

INCLUSION CRITERIA:
1) Children between the age group of 5-9 years of age were selected.
2) Patients with carious lesions either on proximal or occlusal surface of primary molars were included in the study.

3) Only the patients having carious teeth with moderate involvement of dentin (score2/3) according to the radiographic criteria were included in the study (Fig.3)

Criteria used for the radiographic examination for occlusal caries[40]

Score 0 No radiolucency visible
Score 1 Radiolucency visible in the enamel
Score 2 Radiolucency visible in dentin but restricted to the outer third of the dentin.
Score 3 Radiolucency extending to middle third of the dentin.
Score 4 Radiolucency in the pulpal third of the dentin.

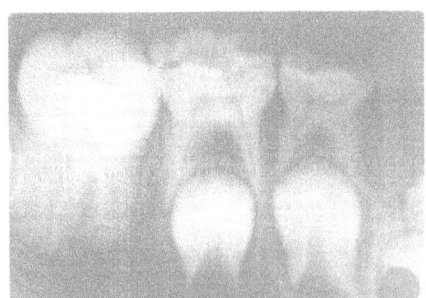

Fig.3: Radiographic examination of occlusal caries

Proximal caries with moderate involvement of dentin (score 3) as confirmed by the radiographic criteria were incorporated in the study. (Fig.4)

Criteria used for radiographic examination of proximal caries[41]

Lesion depth scale
Score 0 Sound

Score 1   Radiolucency in outer half of enamel
Score 2   Radiolucency in inner half of enamel
Score 3   Radiolucency in outer third of dentin.
Score 4   Radiolucency in inner two thirds of dentin

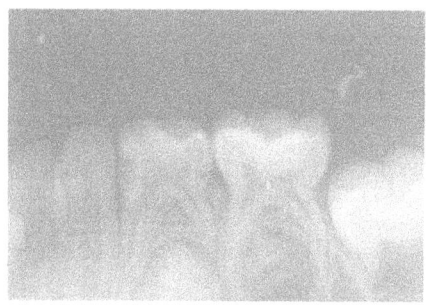

Fig.4: Radiographic examination of proximal caries

1) Only the patients having single surface caries, with no medical history of any systemic diseases and no use of medications were included.
2) Parental consent for the treatment was considered.

EXCLUSION CRITERIA:
1) The carious teeth with the history of spontaneous pain, presence of sinus tract and mobility were excluded from the study.
2) Teeth with extensive (4 score) carious lesions were not considered for the study.

DIVISION OF SAMPLES

A total of 80 patients with sum total of 120 carious teeth fulfilling the inclusion and exclusion criteria were selected for the study and these teeth were designated as samples. These samples were randomly divided in 4 equal groups (Group I to Group IV) based on the method of caries excavation to be employed. The division of samples is further explained as below.

Table 1: Division of samples

Group I (n=30)	Group II (n=30)	Group III (n=30)	Group IV (n=30)
Caries removal by hand instruments	Caries removal by Airotor.	Caries removal by chemomechanical method- Carisolv gel	Caries removal by chemomechanical method– Papacarie

Group I: Caries removal by hand instruments.

This group comprised of 30 carious teeth in which caries excavation was designated to be done using a using sharp spoon excavator.

Group II: By Airotor

30 carious teeth in which the caries was to be removed using number 245 round bur along with adequate coolant were included in group II.

Group III: Caries removal by Carisolv

Carisolv gel was designated to be used in 30 carious teeth which were included in group III.

Group IV: Caries removal by Papacarie

This group comprised of 30 carious teeth in which caries was planned to be removed using Papacarie.

ISOLATION AND APPLICATION OF CARIES DETECTING DYE

The selected tooth was isolated using rubber dam. Caries detecting dye (Caries Detector) containing 1% acid red in propylene glycol was applied using an applicator tip for 10 seconds and was washed with water. After washing with water, carious lesion appeared bright red whereas sound dentin was light pink.

Ericson D et al (1999)[42] scale for assessment of caries:

SCALE 1

0   →   Caries removed completely

1   →   Caries present in base of cavity

2   →   Caries present in base and/ or one wall

3   →   Caries present in base and / or 2 walls

4   →   Caries present in base and / or more than 2 walls

5   →   Caries present in base, walls and margins of cavity

Initial caries was scored according to Ericson D et al scale and was designated as E_0.

EXCAVATION OF CARIES AND CAVITY PREPARATION

Group I: By hand instrument

Following isolation using rubber dam (fig.5a) and application of caries detecting dye (Fig.5b), carious tooth structure was removed using spoon excavators (Hu-friedy) by making circular scooping movements around the long axis of the instrument (Fig.5c)

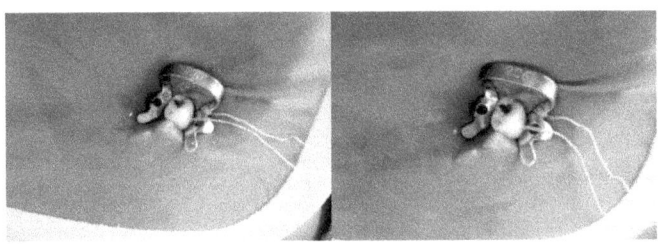

Fig.5a   Fig.5b

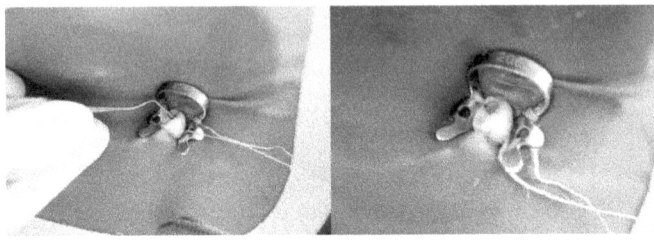

Fig.5c   Fig.5d

Fig.5a: Isolation of carious tooth using rubber dam; 5b: Application of caries detecting dye; 5c: Caries removal using hand instruments; 5d: Application of caries detecting dye after caries removal

After excavation, presence of remaining caries was checked using a sharp probe and caries was excavated till we reached sound dentin. Complete caries removal was finally judged by applying caries detecting dyes again (Fig.5d).

Remaining caries was scored as E_f in accordance with **Ericson D et al scale 1999** [42](mentioned above).

The efficacy of various methods of caries removal was also evaluated in terms of time taken. The time taken from the initial application of caries detecting dye to the subsequent application of dye was recorded as T_H for time taken for caries removal for hand instruments.

The pain felt during the procedure was assessed according to by Visual Analogues Scale[43] (VAS) and Verbal Pain Scale[44].

SCALE 2: Visual Analogue Scale for Pain

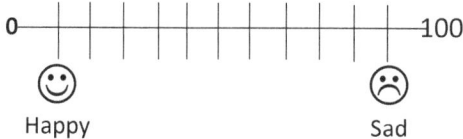

The child was asked to rate the discomfort on a 100 mm visual analogue scale, with a smiling child and one end and a weeping child at the other. The distance along the scale from the smiling child was taken as the pain score and was recorded as VA_H for pain felt during caries removal with hand instruments.

In addition the child was enquired for the pain felt during the procedure and was recorded as Verbal Pain Scale and scored as VP_H for hand instruments.

SCALE 3 - Verbal pain scale

0 → No Pain

1 → Mild pain (Pain recognizable but no discomfort)

2 → Moderate pain (Pain discomforting but bearable)

3 → Severe pain (Pain that causes considerable discomfort and is difficult to bear)

4 → Very severe

If carious dentin was found to be present after the application of the dye, the procedure was repeated until caries removal was complete. This method involved the removal of only carious tooth structure without giving any proper outline form to the cavity.

Group II: Mechanically- using a rotary instrument

Subsequent to isolation using rubber dam (Fig.6a) and application of caries detecting dye (Fig.6b), class I and class II cavity outline form was prepared depending on the extent of caries and Dr. G.V. Black's principles of cavity preparation. Caries was removed using high speed rotary instruments till sound

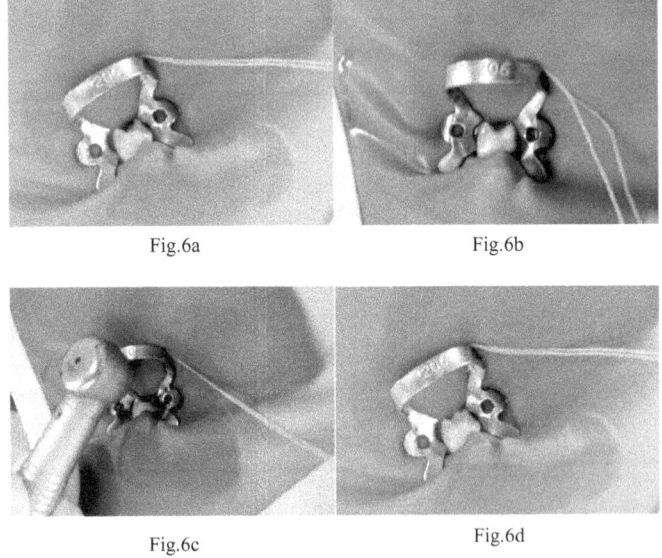

Fig.6a   Fig.6b

Fig.6c   Fig.6d

Fig.6a: Isolation of carious tooth; 6b: Application of caries detecting dye; 6c: Caries removal using Airotor; 6d: Application of caries detecting dye after caries removal

After application of caries detecting dye, the remaining caries was scored E_A in accordance with the **Ericson D et al**[42] scale stated earlier (Fig.6d).

Time taken for caries removal with Airotor, (T_A) was recorded. Pain during the procedure was assessed and recorded as VA_A and VP_A.

Caries removal process was repeated till complete caries removal achieved.

Group III: Chemo-mechanically using Carisolv gel

Following isolation using rubber dam (Fig.7a) and application of caries detecting dye (Fig.7b), access to the lesion was gained if required. The Carisolv gel was mixed using multimix syringe dispenser according to manufacturer's instructions. The mixed gel i.e. the active gel was dispensed onto a mixing well. It was then applied on to the dentinal carious lesion using the hand instrument.

The carious lesion was then covered with the gel. After 60 seconds, the cavity was gently scraped using specialized hand instrument to remove the softened carious tissue (Fig.7c)

On application the gel was clear, but became opaque/ cloudy with debris from the lesion. When the gel was heavily contaminated with debris, it was removed with gentle suction or with a cotton pellet, and fresh gel was applied.

The procedure was repeated until the gel was no longer contaminated with the debris and the surface of the cavity was felt hard. The presence of any remaining caries was checked using a probe. Complete caries removal was judged finally by applying caries detecting dye **Ericson D et al scale (1999)** [42] was used to evaluate the remaining caries and scored as E_F. (Fig.7d)

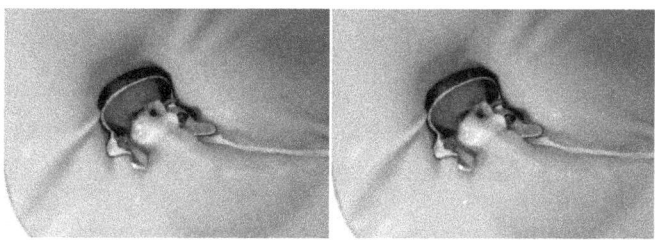

Fig.7a   Fig.7b

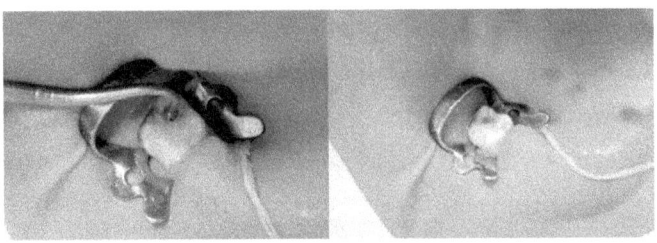

Fig.7c   Fig.7d

Fig.7a:Isolation of carious tooth;7b:Application of caries detecting dye; 7c:Caries removal with specialized hand instruments;7d:Application of caries detecting dye after caries removal

Time taken, T_C was recorded. VAS_C and VPS_C recorded the pain felt during the procedure. If the carious dentin remained, the procedure was repeated until whole caries was removed

Group IV: Caries removal – chemo-mechanically using Papacarie

Following isolation of the tooth using rubber dam (Fig.8a) and application of caries detecting dye (Fig.8b), prophylaxis of the region was first carried out using rubber cup and slurry of pumice. It was followed by rinsing with air/water spray. Access to the lesion was gained. Papacarie was applied using disposable tip attached to the syringe (Fig.8c).The carious lesion was then covered with the gel for 30seconds in acute lesions and for 40-60 seconds in chronic lesions. Initially after application Papacarie was clear. With degradation, oxygen was freed and bubbles appeared on the surface. Blurring of gel was noted. These signs demonstrated that the removal process could be started (Fig.8d).

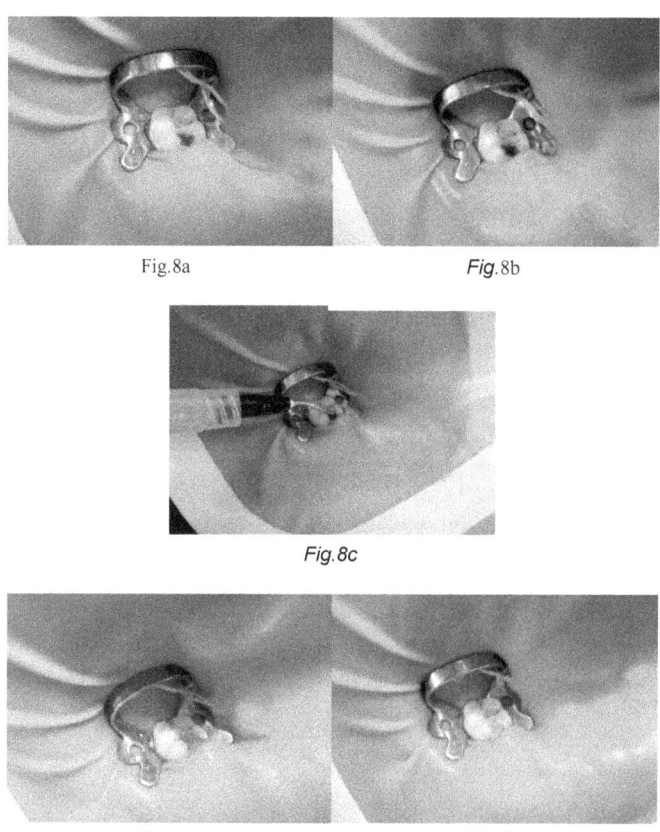

Fig.8a: Isolation of carious tooth; 8b: Application of caries detecting dye; 8c: Application of Papacarie; 8d: Blurring of the gel; 8e: Application of caries detector dye after caries removal

The cavity was gently scraped with hand instruments to remove the softened decayed dentin. The gel was re-applied as many times as necessary, till darkish color appeared, which indicated that decomposition of decayed tissue was still in process. The cavity was not washed in between the application of gel. The procedure was repeated until the gel was no longer contaminated with the debris and the surface of the cavity was felt hard. The presence of any remaining caries was checked using a probe. Caries removal was confirmed finally by applying caries detecting dye and remaining caries was assessed using **Ericson D et al** [42] scale and recorded as E_F mentioned earlier (Fig.8e).

Time taken for the procedure was recorded as T_P. Pain during the procedure was assessed and recorded as VA_P and VP_P.

If the carious dentin was found to be present, the procedure was repeated until the complete caries removal was achieved.

Restoration of the cavity

After the carious dentin was removed, the cavity was restored with Glass Ionomer Cement (GIC Fuji II cement) (Fig.9).

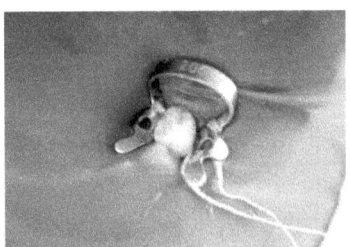

Fig.9: Restoration of cavity

The restorations were checked for occlusal discrepancies using an articulating paper. If any high point was found, it was contoured accordingly using composite finishing burs. After proper occlusion was re-established with no high points, the patients were given post operative instructions.

FLOWCHART SHOWING THE METHODOLOGY

Total number of patients selected = 80
↓
Total number of carious teeth = 120

(Samples)
↓
Application of Caries detecting dye (propylene glycol) applied on carious lesion for 10seconds.
↓
Teeth were randomly divided into four (4) groups according to the method of caries removal

GROUP I	GROUP II	GROUP III	GROUP IV
n=30	n=30	n=30	n=30
Hand instruments	Airotor	Carisolv	Papacarie

↓
Caries detecting dye (propylene glycol) applied on carious lesion for 10seconds.
↓
Washing with water
↓
The efficacy, time taken and the pain threshold was evaluated during the caries removal by **Ericson D et al** scale, visual analogue scale respectively.
↓
Data was collected and statistically analyzed.

OBSERVATIONS & RESULTS

The study was carried out in the out patient Department of Pedodontics and Preventive Dentistry, D.A.V. [C] Dental College & Hospital, Yamuna Nagar. A total number of 120 teeth were included in the study.

The aim of the present study was to compare the efficacy of caries removal by using different methods in children.

The various caries removal methods used were:

1. Caries removal by Hand instruments (Group I)
2. Caries removal by Airotor (Group II)
3. Caries removal by Carisolv (Group III)
4. Caries removal by Papacarie (Group IV)

Statistical Analysis:

The data collected was tabulated and was statistically analyzed using one way analysis of variance (ANOVA) test ad Scheffe Post Hoc Test.

The following statistical formulae were used in the analysis of present study.

1) **MEAN:**

Mean is denoted by $\overline{X}$. It is an effective measure of central tendency and is calculated by dividing the sum of individual observations by the total number of observations i.e.

$$\overline{X} = \frac{\sum x}{N}$$

X = Individual value

Σ = Summation
N = Number of specimens

2) STANDARD DEVIATION:

As every set of data is distributed randomly about the arithmetic mean, the standard deviation is the measure of dispersion of data about its arithmetic mean. It is the root of sum of the squares of the difference of each observation from the mentioned arithmetic mean, divided by total number of values.

Standard deviation is denoted by S.D. = $\sqrt{\dfrac{\sum(X-\overline{X})}{N-1}}$

X = Individual value
$\overline{X}$ = Mean value
N = Number of specimen

3) STANDARD ERROR OF MEAN (S.E.M.):

The magnitude of sampling error and the size of the sample is indicated by the Standard Error of Mean. It indicates the amount of difference anticipated in the observed mean value if a new sample is drawn from the same population. Thus, it may also be called as the Standard deviation of Mean value of a variable when obtained from repeated sample drawn from the same population. S.E.M. = $\dfrac{S.D.}{\sqrt{N}}$

4) To test equality of several means (more than two means)

ANALYSIS OF VARIANCE (ANOVA) was used:

Source of variation	Sum of squares	Degree of freedom	Mean Square
Between Group within group	$SSA = \sum_j \sum ((T.^2 j \ln j) - (T^2 .. 1N))$ $SSW = \sum_j \sum_i x^2 ij - \sum (T.j)^2 \ln j$	K-1 N-k	MSA=SSA / (K-1) MSW=SSW/ N-k)
Total	$SST = \sum_j \sum_i x^2 ij - \dfrac{T^2..}{N}$		

SSW= Sum of squares with in group
The **'p' value** was taken as significant at 'p'< 0.05

5. **Post Hoc Comparisons among Pairs of Means with the Scheffe Test**

In analysis of variance, if F is significant, Scheffe test is applied to see which specific cell mean differs from which other specific cell mean. To do this we calculate an F ratio for the difference between the means of two cells and then test the significance of this F value.

We calculate F_{12} to see if there is a significant difference between the means of groups 1 and 2.

We calculate F_{13} to see if there is a significant difference between the means of groups 1 and 3.

We calculate F_{14} to see if there is a significant difference between the means of groups 1 and 4.

We calculate F_{23} to see if there is a significant difference between the means of groups 2 and 3.

We calculate F24 to see if there is a significant difference between the means of groups 2 and 4.

We calculate F34 to see if there is a significant difference between the means of groups 3 and 4.

The formulas for these tests and their application to the Anova are:

$$F_{12} = \frac{(\bar{X}_1 - \bar{X}_2)^2}{MS_W \left(\frac{1}{n_1} + \frac{1}{n_2} \right)(K-1)}$$

$$F_{13} = \frac{(\bar{X}_1 - \bar{X}_3)^2}{MS_W \left(\frac{1}{n_1} + \frac{1}{n_3} \right)(K-1)}$$

$$F_{23} = \frac{(\bar{X}_2 - \bar{X}_3)^2}{MS_W \left(\frac{1}{n_2} + \frac{1}{n_3} \right)(K-1)}$$

$$F_{23} = \frac{(\bar{X}_2 - \bar{X}_3)^2}{MS_W \left(\frac{1}{n_2} + \frac{1}{n_3} \right)(K-1)}$$

$$F_{23} = \frac{(\bar{X}_2 - \bar{X}_3)^2}{MS_W \left(\frac{1}{n_2} + \frac{1}{n_3} \right)(K-1)}$$

$$F_{23} = \frac{(\bar{X}_2 - \bar{X}_3)^2}{MS_W \left(\frac{1}{n_2} + \frac{1}{n_3} \right)(K-1)}$$

We compare these values with the critical value for $F_{.05}$, and note the significant difference.

A total number of 80 patients were selected from the Out Patient Department of Pedodontics, Preventive and Community Dentistry, D.A.V. (C) Dental College and Hospital, Yamuna Nagar, who presented with single or multiple carious primary teeth. The patients selected had single or multiple primary carious teeth and from these patients a total no. of 120 teeth were selected for the study group (Fig.10). The carious teeth were called as samples and were randomly divided into 4 groups as follows:-

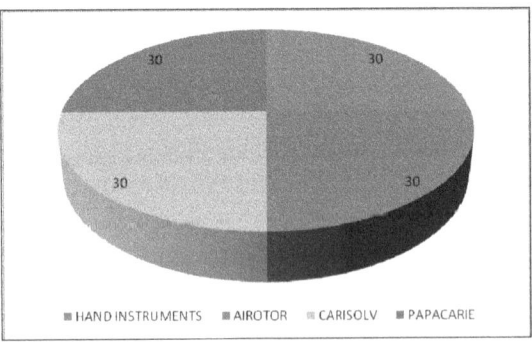

Fig.10: Diagram showing division of samples

TABLE 2: Quantification of mean values of remaining caries (Ericson D et al scale for assessment of efficacy of caries removal)

Name of the method	N	Mean	S.D.	S.E.
Hand instrument	30	2.13	0.900	0.164
Airotor	30	0.27	0.450	0.082
Carisolv	30	0.90	0.845	0.154
Papacarie	30	0.47	0.571	0.104

S.D - standard deviation S.E - standard error

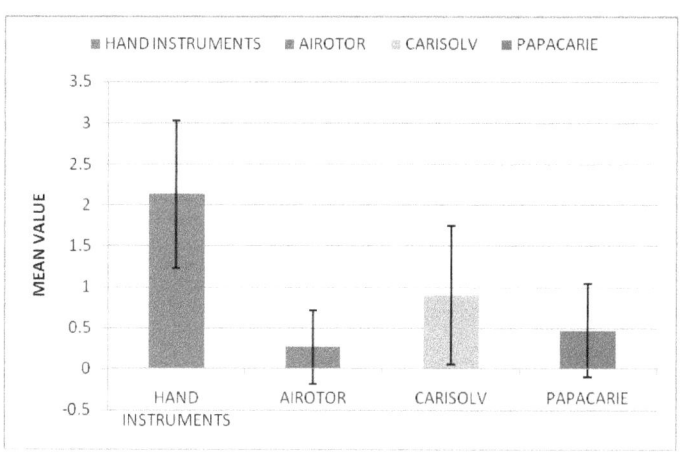

Fig.11: Diagram showing remaining caries following caries removal using different methods

Table 2 depicts mean values of scores of remaining caries illustrating the efficacy of caries removal by different methods, along with statistical derivatives. Remaining caries was observed to be least with Airotor, therefore best efficacy of caries removal was observed with Airotor (0.27 ± 0.450) followed by Papacarie (0.47 ± 0.571), Carisolv (0.90 ± 0.845) and least by the hand instrument technique (2.13 ± 0.9)

TABLE 3: Analysis of variance (ANOVA) for efficacy of caries removal by different methods

	Sum of Squares	Df	Mean Square	F ratio	'p' value	Inference
Between groups	63.092	3	21.031	41.001	0.000[HS]	**Highly Significant**
Within groups	59.500	116	0.513			
Total	122.592	119				

S – Significant , Significant at P < 0.05 ,Not significant (N.S.)

Table 3 shows intergroup comparison of One was Analysis of Variance (ANOVA) of the efficacy of caries removal by using different methods. Highly significant relation ($p<0.05$) were observed when intergroup comparison were made.

TABLE 4: Inter group comparisons of quantified remaining caries (efficacy of caries removal) among experimental groups

Inter group comparisons	Scheffe Post Hoc test		
	Mean Difference	S.E.	'p' Value
Group I Vs II	1.867	0.185	0.000^{HS}
Group I Vs III	1.233	0.185	0.000^{HS}
Group I Vs IV	1.667	0.185	0.000^{HS}
Group II Vs III	-.633	0.185	0.000^{HS}
Group II Vs IV	-.200	0.185	0.760^{NS}
Group III Vs IV	.433	0.185	0.145^{NS}

S- Significant, S.E-Standard error, Significant at P < 0.05,

Non significant results were obtained for the scores observed for efficacy of caries removal when Group IV (Papacarie) was compared with group II (Airotor) and group III (Carisolv). All other intergroup comparisons showed significant results. (Table 4)

TABLE 5: Comparison of mean values of the time taken for caries removal by different methods

Name of the method	N	Mean	S.D.	S.E.
Hand instrument	30	535.83	232.137	42.382
Airotor	30	261.70	86.06	15.712
Carisolv	30	723.73	179.476	32.768
Papacarie	30	590.80	187.004	343.142

S.D- Standard Deviation, S.E- Standard Error

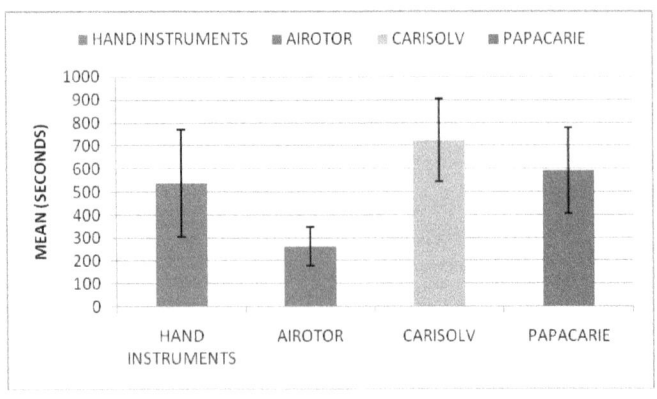

Fig.12: Diagram showing time taken for caries removal using different methods

Table 5 depicts mean values for the time taken for caries removal by different methods along with statistical derivatives. It is observed that among the four methods Airotor removed the caries in minimum time (261.70±86.06seconds), followed by hand instruments (535.83±232.137seconds) and Papacarie (590.80 ±187.004seconds). Carisolv took maximum time for caries removal(723.73±179.476seconds).

Table 6: Analysis of variance values for time taken for removal of caries by different treatment methods.

	Sum of Squares	Df	Mean Square	F Ratio	'p' value	Inference
Between Groups	3396973	3	1132324.27	35.2	0.00	**Highly Significant**
Within Groups	3725817	116	32119.113			
Total	7122790	119				

H.S - Highly significant df - Degree of freedom, Significant at $P < 0.05$

Not significant (N.S.) when $P > 0.05$

Table 6 shows intergroup comparison of One was Analysis of Variance (ANOVA) for the time taken for removal of caries by using different methods. Intergroup comparisons exhibited a highly significant relation ($P<0.05$).

Table 7: Inter group comparisons for time taken among experimental groups for caries removal

Scheffe Post Hoc test			
Inter group comparisons	Mean Difference	S.E.	'p' Value
Group I Vs II	274.133	46.274	0.000^{HS}
Group I Vs III	-187.900	46.274	0.001^{HS}
Group I Vs IV	-54.967	46.274	0.704^{NS}
Group II Vs III	-462.033	46.274	0.000^{HS}
Group II Vs IV	329.100	46.274	0.000^{HS}
Group III Vs IV	329.100	46.274	0.046^{S}

S - Significant, S.E-Standard Error, Significant at P < 0.05,
Not significant (N.S.) when P > 0.05

Non significant results were obtained when Group I & IV (Hand instruments & Papacarie) were compared, whereas all the other groups showed significant results. (Table 7)

TABLE 8: Comparison of mean values of pain using Visual analogue scale (VAS) score for caries removal by different methods

Name of the method	N	Mean	S.D.	S.E.
Hand instrument	30	65.67	11.351	2.7072
Airotor	30	74.00	8.550	1.561
Carisolv	30	19.33	11.725	2.141
Papacarie	30	7.33	5.833	1.065

SD- Standard Deviation, SE- Standard Error

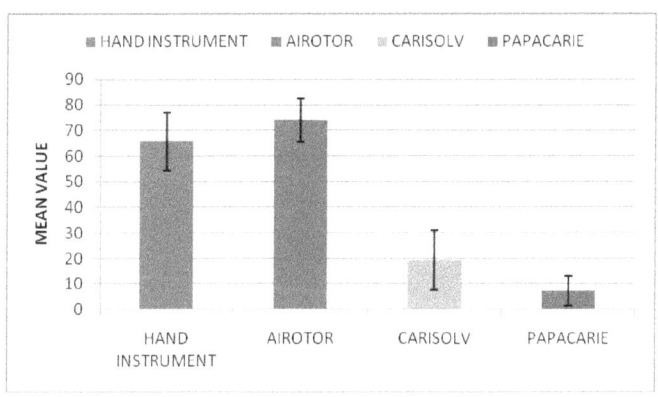

Fig.13: Diagram showing visual analogue scale for pain using different methods of caries removal.

Table 8 depicts mean values for pain using Visual Analogue Scale (VAS) during different methods used in the study for caries removal along with the statistical derivatives. Pain experienced was highest with Airotor (74.00 ± 8.550)

followed by Hand Instruments (65.67 ± 11.351), Carisolv (19.33 ±11.725) and least with Papacarie method (7.33 ± 5.833).

TABLE 9: Analysis of variance (ANOVA) of pain using visual analogue scale (VAS) score among different experimental groups

	Sum of Squares	df	Mean Square	F Ratio	'p' value	Inference
Between Groups	98969.167	3	32989.722	353.353	0.000	**Highly Significant**
Within Groups	10830.000	116	93.362			
Total	109799.2	119				

df - Degree of freedom Significant at P < 0.05 Not significant (N.S.) when P> 0.05

Table 9 shows intergroup comparison of One way Analysis of Variance (ANOVA) of the for pain score as evaluated from the Visual Analogue Scale for different caries removing methods. Highly significant relation (P<0.05) were observed when intergroup comparisons were made.

TABLE 10: Intergroup comparison of pain using Visual analogue scale (VAS) scores among experimental groups

Inter Group comparisons	Scheffe Post Hoc test		
	Mean Difference	S.E.	'p' Value
Group I Vs II	-8.333	2.495	0.013^S
Group I Vs III	46.333	2.495	0.000^{HS}
Group I Vs IV	58.333	2.495	0.000^{HS}
Group II Vs III	54.667	2.495	0.000^{HS}
Group II Vs IV	66.667	2.495	0.000^{HS}
Group III Vs IV	12.000	2.495	0.000^{HS}

Significant at P < 0.05, S.E - Standard Error, Not significant (N.S.) when P > 0.05

All the intergroup comparisons showed highly significant differences.

TABLE 11: Comparison of mean values of pain using verbal scale for all experimental groups

Name of the method	N	Mean	S.D.	S.E.
Hand instrument	30	3.00	.871	.159
Airotor	30	3.40	.724	.132
Carisolv	30	1.93	.868	.159
Papacarie	30	.73	.583	.106

S.D- Standard Deviation S.E-Standard Error

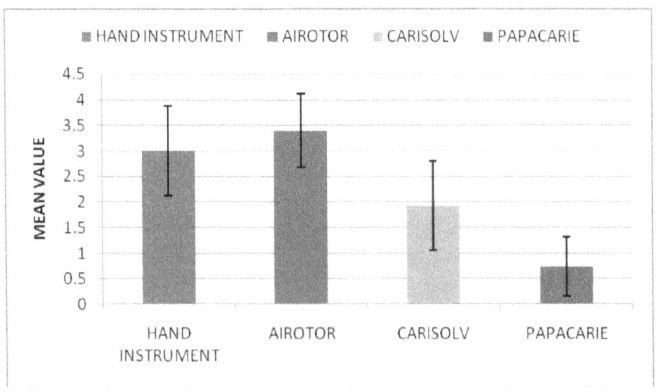

Fig.14: Diagram showing verbal pain using different methods of caries removal.

Table 11 depicts mean values of verbal pain reported by the subjects during caries removal with different methods along with the statistical derivative. Out of the four methods adopted in the present investigation, the mean value of verbal pain score reported by Papacarie method was least (0.73 ± .583) followed by Carisolv method (1.93 ± .868) and hand instruments (3.0 ± .871). Maximum pain was experienced by the subject when caries removal was done with Airotor (3.40±0.724)

TABLE 12: Analysis of variance (ANOVA) for verbal pain during caries removal by different methods

	Sum of Squares	df	Mean Square	F Ratio	'p' value	Inference
Between Groups	128.533	3	42.844	72.098	0.000	**Highly Significant**
Within Groups	68.933	116	.594			
Total	197.467	119				

df - degree of freedom, Significant at P<0.005 ,Not significant (NS) at p >0.005

Table 12 shows intergroup comparison of One way Analysis of Variance (ANOVA) of the for pain score as evaluated from the Verbal pain scale for different caries removing methods. Highly significant relation (P<0.05) were observed when intergroup comparisons were made.

TABLE 13: Intergroup comparison of verbal pain score among different methods used for caries removal

Scheffe Post Hoc test			
Inter Group Comparisons	Mean Difference	S.E.	'p' value
Group I Vs II	-.400	.199	0.263[NS]
Group I Vs III	1.067	.199	0.000[HS]
Group I Vs IV	2.267	.199	0.000[HS]
Group II Vs III	1.467	.199	0.000[HS]
Group II Vs IV	2.667	.199	0.000[HS]
Group III Vs IV	1.200	.199	0.000[HS]

Significant at P < 0.05, S.E-Standard Error, Not significant (N.S.) when P>.05

Non significant results were obtained when group I and II (hand instruments and Airotor) were compared. All other groups showed significant results when intergroup comparisons were made. (Table 13)

DISCUSSION

The word "caries" is derived from the Latin word meaning "rot" and Greek word "ker" meaning death[1]. According to WHO, caries is defined as "localized post erupted, pathological process of external origin involving softening of hard tooth tissue and proceeding to the formation of a cavity."[2]

Dental Caries is a biosocial disease, known to affect the individuals of all age groups, religions, regions, socio-economic status & both the sexes. Both primary and permanent teeth can be affected by the wrath of dental caries and according to the recent oral health survey in India; 50-55% of the population is affected from caries, with an average DMFT of 2.7-3.1. The prevalence is higher in urban areas than in rural and more in girls than in boys[3].

Various efforts for prevention of dental caries are being undertaken at global levels but still it continues to affect a significant portion of the world population. It is asymptomatic in initial stages but may cause discomfort and pain as it progresses. When caries is confined to enamel, various conservative approaches like enameloplasty, atraumatic restorative treatment etc. can be employed. However, once caries progresses to deeper layers of enamel or dentin, the only option left is to excavate the carious tooth structure and to restore it with appropriate restorative material.

The most primitive approach to the treatment of caries was given by Arabian physician Albuscasis who designed specialized hand instruments to scrape away the caries.[45] The early hand instrument with their large heavy handle and inferior metal alloys in the blades, were cumbersome, awkward to use and ineffective in many situations.

To overcome these drawbacks, modern rotary instruments were developed with the manufacturing of powered foot engine patented by **Morrison in 1871**[46].

Due to heavy weight of the drill and low speed, electric motors were introduced. Initially, removal of carious dentin was performed mechanically with the burs in low speed hand pieces (<12000rpm) but in recent years, high speed rotary equipments having approximately 300,000rpm are being used.[4] Exclusive use of high-speed excavation with air turbine hand pieces removes both infected and non-infected dentin, which may cause an excessive cutting and unnecessary weakness of the tooth structure, and may also increase the possibilities of damaging pulpal tissue.[8]

Till recent past, silver amalgam was the material of choice for restoration of cavitated lesion. Cavity preparation for silver amalgam was based on **Dr. G.V. Black's** principle of "Extension for Prevention" resulting in excessive cutting for mechanical retention (**Sturdevant**).[6]

Lately, with the introduction of new adhesive restorative materials, various minimal invasive techniques have been developed, with the aim of removing only carious lesions and maximum preservation of healthy tooth structure. These included air abrasion, sonoabrasion, ultrasonic instrumentation, lasers and chemo-mechanical approach of caries removal[7].

Kinetic energy, applied in the form of micro air-abrasion, follows the path of least resistance, seeking out unsound tooth structure and exposing the underlying decay. Thus, only infected tooth structure is removed, leaving out the healthy part. But, this method is costly, technique sensitive and time consuming which limits its frequent use[5].

Recently, laser technology is introduced which removes both hard and soft carious tissue. It is a safe and effective method for caries removal[5]. But, the cost effectivity and technique sensitivity limits the frequent use of this method. So, the focus was shifted to the use of chemomechanical system which is a cheaper and painless method for caries removal. The procedure involved the application of a chemical solution to the carious dentin followed by gentle removal with hand instruments. This implied minimal removal of sound tooth structure, reduced risk for pulp irritation, less pain and increased patient comfort compared to conventional mechanical methods[47].

Chemomechanical approach is an alternative to traditional drilling. It minimizes sound tissue removal as it is more selective, self limiting, is less painful and prevents permanent damage of dentin layers, by avoiding heating and vibration produced by rotary instruments. The technique softens the pre-degraded collagen of the lesion without undesirable effects to adjacent healthy tissues[7].

In **1975, Habib et al** introduced 5% sodium hypochlorite to remove carious tissue. Since then, many studies have attempted to improve this early method. The sole use of 5% sodium hypochlorite was known to be toxic and aggressive to adjacent healthy tissues[48].Therefore, the first chemo-mechanical caries removal system was introduced in 1975 by a formula, called GK 101, which consisted of N-monochloroglycine (NMG). GK 101 turned out to act slowly and additional efforts to speed up the procedure resulted in GK 101 E. Based on GK 101 E, a caries removal system called Caridex was introduced in **1985** by **Schutzbank et al**[22]. This system was based on non specific proteolytic effect of sodium hypochlorite (NaOCl) which was reacted with an amino acid to reduce the aggressive effect on sound tooth structure[45;50]. A system using N-monochloro-DL-2 aminobutyric acid (NMAB) was developed which involved the chlorination of partially degraded collagen in carious dentin, and the conversion of hydroxyproline to pyrrole-2-carboxylic acid which initiates the disruption of the altered collagen fibres in carious dentin[50].

Despite of its effectiveness, Caridex system had certain clinical limitations including the requirement of large reservoir with pump, large volume of solution needed and short shelf life the prolonged period of time to complete the procedures. **(Beeley JA et al 2000)**[50]

The shortcomings of the Caridex system were addressed in the development of Carisolv by **Ericsson et al**[23] and was introduced in Swedish market in 1997. Carisolv is a minimally invasive method for chemomechanical dentin caries removal and consist of 2 component mixture. One of the components contains 3 aminoacids (glumatic acid, lysine leucine), 0.1 M. The other transparent liquid containing 0.5% sodium hypochlorite[9]. When the gel and fluid are mixed, amino acids bind chlorine and form chloramines at a pH of 11.These amino acids counteract aggressive behaviour of sodium hypochlorite to the oral healthy tissues. The result of these processes is breakdown of degraded collagen found in demineralized portion of a carious lesion[9,23]. The degraded collagen has an open structure and is, therefore, more susceptible to further breakdown by chloramines. The porous nature of demineralized dentin allows penetration of Carisolv. The unaffected collagen is more resistant to degradation but the framework of degraded collagen is broken down and can be easily scraped away[23]. Therefore Carisolv removes caries selectively by reacting with the denatured collagen thereby making carious dentin soft without affecting healthy dentin[51].

Inspite of its effectiveness and various advantages, Carisolv^{TM} is not globally accepted as it required an extensive training, use of customised instruments, an increased cost and limited availability[10].

Therefore, in 2003 a research project in Brazil led to the development of a new formula to universalize the use of chemo-mechanical method for caries removal and to promote its use in public health. This new formula was commercially known as Papacarie. It composed of papain, chloramine and toluidine blue was launched to be used as chemomechanical caries removal method[10].

Papain is an endoprotien, with bacteriostatic, bactericidal and anti-inflammatory activity[10,52,53,54]. Chloramines, contains chlorine and ammonia, possessing bactericidal and disinfectant properties which is used to irrigate root canals and to chemically soften carious dentin. The degraded portion of carious dentin collagen is chlorinated by the solution, which helps in chemical and mechanical caries removal[10].

Papain acts as a debridement anti inflammatory agent which does not damage the healthy tissue and accelerates the cicatricial process. Papain facilitates the cleansing of both necrotic tissues and secretions. As a result, it decreases the time required for tissue recovery and does not damage the sound tissues around the lesion.

According to **Mandelbaum 2003**[53], Papain is indicated in all phases of the cicatricial process; dry or exudative wounds, colonised or infected, with or without areas of necrosis. Papain promotes chemical debridement, granulation and epithelialization, which hastens the phases of cicatrization and stimulation of the tensile strength of the scars.

When the treatment with papain is initiated it increases the local reparative secretion, softens the necrotic tissue, slacks the borders of the lesion and promotes a small increase in hyperaemic halo diameter. A period after the beginning of the process, the necrotic tissue breaks loose and the hyperemic halo diameter slowly starts to decrease. Therefore, the cicatricial process is accelerated, which reduces the time required for the recovery of the patients lesion. The topical use of papain softens scabs of lesions and can cause borders to break loose[10].

Flindt et al 1979[55] demonstrated that papain acts only in infected tissues because tissues lack a plasmatic anti-protease called a1-anti-tyrpsin. The a1-anti-tyrpsin is only present in the sound tissues and it inhibits protein digestion. The absence of a1-anti-tyrpsin in infected tissues allows papain to break the partially degraded collagen molecules.

Papain comes from the latex of the leaves and fruits of the green adult papaya[10]. **Dawkins** showed that Carica papaya has bactericide and bacteriostatic properties. He investigated antibacterial activity of ripe and unripe Carica papaya on selected micro-organisms. They concluded that the Carica papaya contain anti-bacterial activity that inhibits growth of gram positive and gram-negative organisms[56].

Chloramines another component of Papacarie are formed during the reaction between chlorine and ammonia. Chloramines are amines which contain at least one atom chlorine atom, which is directly bonded to nitrogen atoms. They have bactericidal and disinfectant properties. Chloramines are broadly used to chemically soften the carious dentin[10]. According to **Maragakis et al 2001**[57] the partially degraded collagen in carious dentin was chlorinated by chemo-mechanical caries removal solutions. This chlorination affects the secondary and/or quaternary structure of the collagen, by disrupting hydrogen bonding and thus facilitating the carious tissue removal.

Application of chloramines resulted in the opening of dentinal tubules in the outer layer of carious dentin and occluded dentinal tubules were seen after sodium hypochlorite application. The presence of chloramines and amino acids had some effect on the carious dentin outer layer. However, chloramines activity was supposed to be influenced by the pH of the solution, types of amino acids and proportion of amino acids and sodium hypochlorite. **(Tonami 2003)**[58].

Before the clinical use of Papacarie several in vitro and in vivo studies were undertaken to validate its safety in clinical procedures[10]. Papacarie is safe, not cytotoxic in vitro fibroblast culture and is biocompatible to the oral tissues. **(Silva et al 2003)**[59]. Papacarie has antimicrobial properties, with maximum activity against streptococcus and lactobacillus **(Pereira et al)**[60].

Study conducted by **Reda et al**[61] among professionals and graduate students verified Papacarie's effectiveness, action time, consistency, oxygen liberation and patient symptom and it showed that gel showed fast action, ideal consistency, effectiveness, no sensitivity and almost no bubbling during the oxygen liberation.

Mechanism of action of Papacarie: Anti-trypsin inhibits protein digestion but infected tissues do not usually show anti-tyrpsin. Since papain can digest only dead cells, it acts breaking the partially degraded collagen molecules, contributing to the degradation and elimination of the fibrin "mantle" formed by the carious process. Papain gel breaks the bonds between fibres of carious dentin collagen, leaving intact dentin. It acts only on denatured collagen fibres due to its proteolytic action and through chlorination of ultrastructural collagen fibres. This is the reason why the gel has no effect on the healthy tissue, either dentin or pulp[10].

After the degradation, oxygen is freed, bubbles appear on the surface, and a blearing of the gel is thus noted. These signs demonstrate that the removal process can be started. The instrument should scrap the carious tissue without promoting any kind of stimulus or pressure[10].

According to the manufacturer, the product is indicated for deep carious lesions and root caries, for caries removal that requires no application of local anaesthesia or use of rotary cutting instruments. The gel can be used in periodontology for the chemical – mechanical treatment of the root surface facilitating the removal of calculus and smoothening the root[62].

Despite the availability of various methods and materials for caries removal, the most preferable method of caries removal in paediatric patients would be the one which is painless and which effectively removes soft carious tooth structure without causing pain.

Regardless of the fact that the newer chemo-mechanical methods of caries removal are comfortable and acceptable, there is still lack of adequate clinical studies comparing their efficacy and adequacy with conventional methods for caries removal in paediatric patients. Therefore, the present study was undertaken to compare the clinical efficacy of chemo-mechanical caries removal with conventional caries removal methods in children.

Eighty patients with a sum total of 120 carious teeth, between the age group of 5-9 years were selected from the Out Patient Department of Pedodontics, Preventive and Community Dentistry, D.A.V (c) Dental College and Hospital, Yamuna Nagar. The teeth with the history of pain and/or presence of sinus tract were not included in the study. Only those teeth with moderate involvement of dentin (score 2/3 for occlusal caries (**Ricketts DNJ et al 2002**)[40] and score 3 for proximal caries (**Hintze H et al 1998**)[41], which were judged according to radiographic criteria were selected for the study.

Children between age group 5-9 years were selected for the study as caries incidence shows three peaks at ages 4-8years, 11-19 years and between 55 and 65 years. (**Niki Foruk**)[63]. Also, according to **Mariri 2003**[64] caries activity is high during this age group due to increased intake of sugars, starchy foods and greater frequency of eating. In this age group patient responses are also well developed which leads to easy communication between the child and the dentist. Also this is an appropriate age till which primary molars must be preserved. A study was done by **Mugonzibwa EA et al 2002**[65] which showed that the primary molars do not shed in 6 - 9 years of age. So, the tooth should be restored during this period with all possible efforts.

Children less than 5 year of age were not included in the study because, only the children over 5 years of age are able to use self assessment pain scales like the visual analogue scale in a reliable and valid manner to describe their perceptions. (**Mc Granth A 1987**) [66]

A total number of 80 patients with a sum total of 120 carious teeth were selected for the study. These teeth were designated as samples and were randomly divided into four groups (with 30 samples in each group) according to the caries removal method to be followed:

Group I: Caries removal by Hand instruments
Group II: By Airotor
Group III: Caries removal by Carisolv
Group IV: Caries removal by Papacarie

In Group I, the selected carious teeth were isolated using rubber dam and the initial caries was scored E_0 according to **Ericson D et al**[42] **scale 1999**, after the application of caries detecting dye. Carious tooth structure was removed following the technique described in **ART manual**[67] that is by making circular scooping movements around the long axis using spoon excavators (Hu-friedy).

After excavation, presence of remaining caries was checked using a sharp probe and caries was excavated till we reached sound dentin. Complete caries removal was finally judged by applying caries detecting dyes again and the remaining caries was scored as E_f according with **Ericson D et al**[42] scale.

In Group-II the carious teeth were isolated with rubber dam and initial caries was scored following the application of caries detecting dye. The access was gained with a round bur. The cavity preparation was done according to Dr. G.V. Black's principle which included a proper outline form, resistance, retention form, and an adequate depth. After the caries was removed, caries detecting dye (propylene glycol based dye) was applied on the cavity using applicator tip. The cavity was washed and extent of caries removal was seen visually and remaining caries was scored. **Vande Rijke 1991 et al**[49] also used hardness, texture of tissue, colour and caries detecting dye to clinically evaluate the caries removal status. **Ericson D et al 1999**[23], **Kakaboura et al 2003**[68] also removed the caries in the same way as was done in the present study.

In Group-III the selected carious teeth were isolated using rubber dam. Initial caries was scored following the action of Papacarie. Caries was removed by using Carisolv. The Carisolv gel is a two component mixture. Equal parts of the two components are mixed to form an active gel substance. The mixed gel i.e. the active gel was dispensed onto a mixing well. It was then applied on to the dentinal carious lesion using specially designed hand instruments. The carious lesion was then covered with the gel. After 60 seconds, the cavity was gently scraped using specialised hand instruments to remove the softened carious tissue. This was done in accordance with the procedure followed by **Munshi AK et al 2001**[9].

Similar procedure was followed **Balciuniene I et al 2005**[31] and **Chourio MAL et al 2006**[33].

On application the gel was clear, but became opaque/cloudy with debris from the lesion. When the gel was heavily contaminated with debris, it was removed with gentle suction or with a cotton pellet, and fresh gel was again applied.

The procedure was repeated until the gel was no longer contaminated with the debris and the surface of the cavity was felt hard. The cavity was checked using a probe (DG -16). Complete caries removal was judged by applying caries detecting dye (propylene glycol). If the caries dentin remained, the procedure was repeated.

In Group IV following isolation using rubber dam and application of caries detecting dye, prophylaxis of the region was first carried out using rubber cup and slurry of pumice. It was followed by rinsing with air/water spray. Access to the lesion was gained.

Papacarie was applied according to manufacturer's instructions and the carious lesion was then covered with the gel for 30seconds in acute lesions and for 40-60 seconds in chronic lesions. After application Papacarie was clear initially. Later on with degradation, oxygen was freed and bubbles appeared on the surface and blurring of gel was noted. These signs demonstrated that the caries removal process was started. **(Bussadori SK et al 2005)**[10]

The cavity was gently scraped with hand instruments to remove the softened decayed dentin. The gel was re-applied as many times as necessary, till dark colour appeared, which indicated that decomposition of decayed tissue was still in process. The cavity was not washed in between the application of gel. The procedure was repeated until the gel was no longer contaminated with the debris and the surface of the cavity was felt hard. The presence of any remaining caries was checked using a probe. Caries removal was confirmed finally by applying caries detecting dye and remaining caries was assessed using **Ericson D et al scale1999**[42] and recorded.

If the carious dentin was found to be present, the procedure was repeated until the complete caries removal was achieved. After the carious dentin was removed, the cavity was restored with Glass Ionomer Cement (GIC Fuji II cement) according to **Burrow MF et al 2002**[25].

The above mentioned procedures were evaluated for their efficacy of caries removal, time taken to remove caries by each method and the pain perception by the respective procedure, by using the following scales:

1. Scale to check the efficacy of caries removal **(Ericsson D et al 1999)**[9,42].
2. Time scale **(Munshi AK et al)**[9]
3. Pain Scales
a) Visual Analogue Scale **(Huskinson EC 1974)**[43]
b) Verbal Pain Scale **(Keele 1976)**[44]

I. Efficacy of caries removal:

Efficacy of caries removal can be evaluated both by in vivo and in vitro methods. In invitro, the extent of caries removal have been judged by histological sections **(Fluckiger et al 2005)**[30], micro-hardness **(Magalhes CS et al 2006)**[47], autofluorescence assessment using SEM **(Banerjee A et al 2000)**[5], electrical caries monitor **(Moran et al 2000)**[5] etc. While clinically, ths efficacy of caries removal have been evaluated by visual criteria **(Fure S et al 2004)**[69], tactile sensation **(Ericsson D et al 1999)**[23,42] and by caries detecting dyes **(Ziskind D et al)**[70]. Various scales that can be used for the assessment of caries removal are **Ericsson D et al 1999**[23,42] scale and **Bornstein et al**[5] scale. In the present study **Ericsson D et al**[23,42] scale was used as it was found to be is more descriptive and simple to use. **Bornstein et al scale**[5] does not described the extent of caries removed.

II. Time Scale

For the convenience of the clinician the time taken was divided into groups according to different studies done. In this study the time scale taken was in accordance with the time scale taken by **Munshi AK et al 2001**[10].The time taken for removal of carious dentin, beginning from the application of the gel until the completion of the procedure was evaluated using stopwatch.

III. Assessing Pain

Various pain assessment scales are available like Visual Analogue Scale, Numeric pain intensity scale, Graphic rating scale, Verbal pain scale, Pain faces scale etc. Of these Visual analogue scale and Verbal pain scale were used in the present study.

a)   Visual Analogue Scale:

Visual Analogue Scale was originally developed by **Huskisson EC et al 1974**[71]. It is a gold standard for assessment of pain in communicating patients. According to **Mc Grath PA 1987**[66], Visual Analogue Scale for Pain is reliable and valid manner to describe the perception of pain of a child as young as 6 years of age. It enables the patients to identify and express emotions easily and quickly[36]. The VAS method has a potential utility for measurement of a variety of clinical procedure. (**Wewers ME et al 1990**)[71]. It is demonstrated to be reliable (**Price et al 1983, 1987; Wade et al 1990**)[72], generalizable (**Price and Harkins 1987**)[73]. According to **Versloot et al 2005**[74] Visual Analogue Scale is useful for acquiring into behavioural aspects of young children as a consequence of dental treatment, thereby identifying the importance of a behavioural approach in young children.

b)   Verbal Pain Scale :

Verbal pain scale was first described by **Keele**[75] in **1948.** According to **Rafique S et al 2003**[27.] Verbal Pain Scale is a best method for scaling different dimensions of pain experienced by an individual.

Thus, in our study this scale was used as it was simple, descriptive and more informative about the type of pain. The data was collected and statistically analysed using ANOVA and Post hoc test.

1. **Efficacy of caries removal:**

    The mean value of remaining caries by Group I, Hand instrument was observed to be 2.13 while that of Group II, Airotor showed a mean value of 0.27. Caries remaining in Group III, Carisolv showed mean value of 0.90. Finally the mean value of Group IV Papacarie was 0.47.

    There was a highly significant difference ($p<0.05$) in efficacy of caries removal when intergroup comparison were made.

    These results indicated that the efficacy of caries removal was highest with Airotor followed by almost comparable Papacarie method followed by Carisolv and least by the Hand instrument.

    The results were in accordance to the study by **Banerjee et al 2000**[51] which showed that effectiveness of caries removal was the highest with Airotor, however least efficacy was exhibited by Carisolv. The studies done by **Ericsson D et al (1999)**[23,42], **Watson et al (2000)**[49], **Fure S et al (2000)**[69] had also concluded that the Carisolv was as effective as bur in removing infected dentin. However, **Yazici AR et al 2003**[28] showed success rate in only 36% of cases treated with Carisolv.

    The efficacy of removing caries with Airotor was the highest because it tends to over prepare the cavities due to lack of sensitivity of tactile feedback. This resulted in gross rapid removal of tissue with reduced control over the whole process. Thus, it was not always apparent to the operator when the true clinical end point was reached. So, the excavation procedure continued in healthier dentin leading to eventual over preparation[49].Carbide or diamond bur used with high speed for cavity preparation often remove reversibly affected dentin along with the odontoblastic reaction zone plugs, resulting in the exposure of the more permeable healthy dentin [58].

Papacarie, a chemo-mechanical caries removal technique showed clinical efficacy almost comparable to Airotor. Study by **Calvo et al 2005**[76] showed that papain gel enables effective carious tissue removal without causing troubles in patients. Also study by **Torices S et al 2007**[77] reported Papacarie an efficient technique for caries removal in children.

Thus, Carisolv removes the soft irreversibily damaged, highly infected dentinal tissue, while conserving the reversely affected dentin. **Splieth et al (2001)**[78,] evaluated the remaining caries with methyl red dye, and reported that the chemomechanical caries removal leaves about 50µm more carious dentin than round burs. Caries affected dentin is useful because of its low permeability compared to healthy dentin, which protects the pulp from any remaining bacteria.

Whereas, **Maragakis et al (2001)**[24] reported that the efficacy of caries removal by Carisolv was only 62.5% showing that it did not remove the caries efficiently and therefore cannot replace the rotary instruments. The amount of residual caries dentin did not differ significantly between hand excavation and Carisolv. (**Fluckiger L et al 2005**)[30]. **Peters MC et al 2006**[32] concluded that chemomechanical caries removal had lower efficacy and efficiency when treating dentinal depth occlusal lesions with minimal opening in primary molars than traditional methods.

93% of teeth showed complete removal of caries whereas chemomechanically prepared teeth showed only 36% of caries removal. The results of this study suggest that conventional rotary instrument (bur) was more effective than Carisolv in removal of carious tissue and also takes shorter time.

Earlier studies showed high rates of chemomechanical caries removal from 94 -100%, which was judged using a dental explorer (14,20,26/0. In a more reproducible approach, **Moran et al (1999)**[24], evaluated the caries removal using an electric caries monitor, which resulted in similar values for chemomechanical treatment and conventional caries removal with a round bur. **Banerjee et al (2000)**[5] reported similar auto fluorescence readings for chemomechanical treatment.

Numerous studies have reported the effectiveness and clinical safety of chloramines gel and concluded that patients felt no discomfort during the treatment and therefore this gel is a promising material for the treatment of primary teeth and being more comfortable than conventional method. **(Anusavice KJ et al**[79]**)**[10, 80,81,82,83,34]

II. Time Scale

The time taken for the complete caries removal was calculated, from the start of the procedure to the completion of caries removal. The results obtained showed that the mean value of time taken for caries removal by Carisolv method was found to be maximum 723.73 seconds followed by caries removal with Papacarie gel, 590.80seconds. Mean value for hand instruments used for caries removal was 535.83 seconds followed by Airotor method, 261.70 seconds.

Thus it is observed that among the four methods Airotor removed the caries in the minimum time. The results of this study showed that the primary molars treated with chemomechanical technique needed significantly more time for caries removal than the primary molars treated with Airotor. This was in accordance with the study conducted by **Banerjee et al (2001)**[5] who evaluated 5 alternative methods (bur, air abrasion, sonoabrasion, Carisolv, hand instruments) of carious dentin excavation and found that Airotor was the quickest method and Carisolv excavation was slowest out of the five methods. They also observed that the Airotor tends to over prepare the cavities whereas Carisolv only removed infected dentin. Thus, it was concluded, that even though Carisolv was a time consuming method, but, it removed the caries effectively.

Torices SS et al 2007[77] showed work time acceptability in paediatric dentistry. The time ranged between 4 to 8 min. The time spent for the removal of caries in Papacarie system and in hand excavation method was (10.9±4.46 min) and (7.87±2.92 min) respectively (**Barata TJE 2008**)[83]. Papacarie gel had a completed caries removal time of 8 minutes per tooth **(Carrillo C M 2008)**[37].

The mean value of time taken for caries removal by Carisolv method was observed to be maximum 723.73 ± 179.476 seconds followed by Papacarie (590.80 ± 187.004 seconds), Hand instrument method (535.83 ± 232.137 seconds) and Airotor method (261.70 ± 80.06 seconds) respectively. Highly significant relation was found ($p<0.05$) when intergroup comparisons were made. According to the study done by **Kakaboura et al 2003**[68] the reason for increased time taken by Carisolv might be because of the multiple applications of Carisolv gel for complete caries removal. They also stated that when the Carisolv gel was applied on the carious lesion it was clear, but it became opaque/ cloudy with debris from the lesion. When the gel was heavily contaminated with debris, it was removed with a cotton pellet and fresh gel was again applied. The procedure was repeated until the gel was no longer contaminated with debris. Thus, multiple applications of Carisolv gel led to increased time taken to remove caries by Carisolv. However, **Lennon AM et al 2006**[85] reported time taken for caries removal with chemomechanical methods to be only 5 minutes.

Bergmann et al 2005[86] reported that the time spent for caries removal with chemomechanical method was significantly higher than hand piece. Similar results were observed with a study reported by **Pandit et al 2007**[34]. Operative time with the chemomechanical method was much longer than the conventional method, but this did not adversely affect the cooperation of children (**Kavvadias K et al 2004**)[87].

Chourio MAL et al (2006)[33] demonstrated that the time spent for chemical-mechanical caries removal was three times longer than the conventional method with Airotor method.

Ericson D et al (1999)[23,42] reported the mean caries removal time was 10.40 min with Carisolv and 4.42 min with rotary instruments. This is comparable with the treatment time found in the present study. Similar results were seen in the studies of **Maragakis et al 2001**[24] and **Fure et al 2000**[69].

III. For Assessing Pain:

a) **Visual Analogue Scale**

This scale was used in various clinical studies done by **Allen KL et al 1999**[88], **Anusavice et al 1987**[79], **Rafique S et al 2003**[27].

The observations of visual analogue scale differed significantly between the groups. The mean value of VAS score in Group-I (Hand Instrument) was observed to be 65.67 and in Group-II (Airotor) was 74.00. While the mean value for VAS score in Group-III (Carisolv) was 19.33 and Group IV (Papacarie) was 7.33. Thus the pain experienced was found to be maximum with Airotor followed by Hand Excavation and Carisolv and the least by Papacarie.

The results were in accordance with **Barata TJE et al**[84] who compared Papacarie and to atraumatic restorative treatment for pain using Visual analogue scale. Results showed that 72 % patients presented with no pain during the treatment.

Patients' acceptance was assessed using the visual analogue scale. The visual scale was presented

Anusavice and Kinchloe (1987)[79] demonstrated that cutting or removing carious dentin generally elicits little or no sensation, while cutting sound dentin often results in some level of pain and sensitivity. This has been the basis of the clinical evaluation of the chemomechanical method of caries removal. Similar data have been presented in the studies of **Zinck et al (1988)**[89,23,42,27,69,34].

The unpleasant sensation of scraping the decay with hand excavation and the vibration associated with the use of Airotor during caries removal makes the treatment more traumatic than chemomechanical caries removal system[27]. Rotary instruments are universal method of caries removal but pain and discomfort are associated with the cavity preparation, due to sensitivity of vital pulp, pressure in the tooth (eg. mechanical stimulus), conduction of noise and vibration to the bone, sharp noise and finally due to development of high temperatures on the surface cut due to thermal stimulation. The Carisolv gel is effective only on the denuded fibres in the demineralized dentin, thus painful removal and damage to sound dentin is avoided[90]. Also the gel itself has a thermal insulating properties as it covers the cavity during the procedure, and hence leads to less pulpal stimulation. According to **Braum et al**[5] slight anaesthetic effect from the gel has also been observed.

A study was conducted by **Fiske J et al (2002)**[27] to investigate whether caries removal with Carisolv gel/air abrasion is an alternative to conventional local anaesthetics and drills in the treatment of patients. They used Visual Analogue Scale to assess the pain using different methods of caries removal. The conclusion was that air abrasion /Carisolv treatment was a well accepted and viable alternative to conventional local anaesthetics and drill for dental patients.

Bergemann J et al 2005[86] compared patient acceptance against two chemo-mechanical and traditional method (handpiece). Significantly lower degree of pain was experienced when caries was removed using chemomechanical caries removal method and hence more patient acceptance was found with chemo-mechanical method.

b) **Verbal Pain Scale:**

The mean value of verbal pain score reported by the subjects was observed to be 0.73 for Papacarie method for caries removal, followed by Carisolv (1.93), hand instruments (3.00) and Airotor (3.40). Thus, it is derived that out of all the methods adopted in the present investigation, Papacarie method seems to be least painful with respect to caries removal.

Highly significant relation was found (P<0.05) when intergroup comparisons were made between hand instruments and Carisolv/Papacarie and Airotor and Carisolv/Papacarie. Comparison of Airotor group with Hand Instrument and Carisolv and Papacarie group did not demonstrate any significant difference.

The results were similar to those as observed by **Gurbuz T et al 2004**[91] who concluded in a study that chemo-mechanical method was an effective method in removal of caries causing less pain and need for local anaesthesia , thus decreasing fear ,anxiety and stress of children.

Papain interacts with exposed collagen by the dissolution of dentin minerals through bacteria, making the infected dentin softer, and allows its removal with non-cutting instruments without local anaesthesia and burs (**Bussadori SK et al 2008**)[10].

Banerjee et al 2000[49] stated that the reason for mild pain experienced in Group-III (Carisolv) and Group IV (Papacarie) was because of the prolonged time taken to remove the caries. **Calvo et al 2005**[76] showed that papain gel enabled effective caries removal without causing pain in patients.

Singh KA et al 2000[92] concluded from a study that invasive dental treatment increases the anxiety level in children and therefore induces a negative behaviour in children. Similar results were observed by **Chourio MAL et al (2006)**[33]. Pain was reported during caries removal with high speed rotary instruments (**Pandit et al 2007**)[34].

Hence, based on the observations obtained in the present study, it was concluded that out of all the methods used for caries removal Papacarie proved to be an effective, virtually painless and non invasive technique of caries removal.

Thus, it appears to be of potential interest for use especially in clinical pediatric dentistry.

CONCLUSION

The present study was undertaken to clinically evaluate the different methods of caries removal in children. The caries was removed by using different methods such as hand instruments, airotor, carisolv and papacarie.

Children between age group of 5-9 years were selected for the study and were randomly divided into four groups according to the caries removal method followed. The efficacy of caries removal, time taken to remove caries by each method and the pain reflected upon the respective procedure was recorded by using **Ericsson D. et al** scale for Efficacy of Caries Removal, Time scale, Visual Analogue Scale (VAS) and Verbal Pain Scale. The data collected was tabulated and statistically analyzed. The following conclusions were drawn from the study:

1. All the four methods removed caries effectively, however, the efficacy of caries removal using **Ericsson et al scale** was highest with Airotor followed by almost comparable effectiveness by Papacarie and Carisolv method and the least by the hand instruments.
2. The time taken to remove caries by Carisolv method was observed to be significantly higher followed by Papacarie and hand instrument method. Minimum time was taken by Airotor method.
3. The pain experienced by the patients during caries removal was found to be significantly higher with Airotor followed by Hand Excavation and then Carisolv and least pain was experienced when Papacarie method was used.
4. The chemomechanical removal of caries with Papacarie and Carisolv were found to be effective measures and could be considered as viable alternatives to painful procedures like Airotor in management of dental caries especially in children.

REFRENCES

1. **Tandon S**. Dental caries in early childhood. Textbook of Pedodontics. 1st edition. Paras publishing 2003.p.178-210.
2. **Sikiri VK**. Dental caries. Textbook of Operative Dentistry. 2nd edition. CBS publishers & distributors. 2008. p.40-60.
3. WHO india .org/ link files / oral health- multicentric
4. **Bayne SC, Thompson JY, Sturdevant CM, Taylor DF.** Instruments and equipment for tooth preparation. In: **Roberson TM, Heymann HO, Swift EJ.** Editors. Art & Science of Operative Dentistry. 4th edition. Mosby publications; 2002.p.307-345.
5. **Banerjee A, Kidd EAM, Watson TF.** In vitro evaluation of five alternative methods of carious dentine excavation. Caries Research 2000; 34: 144-150
6. **Roberson TM, Sturdevent CM.** Fundamentals in Tooth Preparation. In: **Roberson TM, Heymann HO, Swift EJ**. Editors .Art & Science of Operative Dentistry. 4th edition. Mosby publications; 2002.p.271-306.
7. **Beeley JA, Yip HK, Stevenson AG**. Chemomechanical caries removal: A review of the techniques and latest developments. Br. Dent J 2000; 34: 144-150.
8. **Correa FNP, Rocha RDO, Filcho LER, Rodrigues CRMD**. Chemical versus conventional caries removal techniques in primary teeth: A microhardness study. J Clin Pediatr Dent 31(3): 189-194, 2007.
9. **Munshi AK, Hegde AM, Shetty PK**. Clinical evaluation of carisolv in chemo-mechanical removal of carious dentin. J Clin Pediatr Dent 26(1): 49-54, 2001.
10. **Bussadori SK, Castro LC, Galvao AC**. Papain gel: A new chemo-mechanical caries removal agent. J Clin Pediatr Dent 30(20): 115-120, 2005.

11. **Schricks MCM, Amerongen WL.** Atraumatic Perspective of ART: psychological and physiological aspects of treatment with and without rotary instruments. Community Dent Oral Epidemol 2003; 31: 15-20.
12. **Lopez N, Rafalin SS, Berthold P.** Atraumatic Restorative treatment for Prevention and Treatment of Caries in an underserved community. Am J Public Health. 2005 August; 95(8): 1338-1339.
13. **Frencken JE, Holmgren CJ.** ART: a minimal intervention approach to manage dental caries. Dent Update 2004. June ; 31 (5) : 295-8,301.
14. **Deery C.** Atraumatic Restorative Techniques could reduce discomfort in children receiving dental treatment. Evidence based dentistry 2005.6;9
15. **Ersin, Kocatas N, Uzel, Atacb, Aykut, Arzu A et al.** Inhibition of Cultivable Bacteria by Chlorhexidine. Treatment of dentin lesions treated with the ART technique. Caries Res 2006, 40:2.
16. **Toi CS, Bonecker M, Jones PEC.** Mutans streptococci strains prevalence before and after cavity preparation during Atraumatic Restorative Treatment .Oral Microbiology and Immunology. 2009. Vol 18, issue 3; p.160-164.
17. **Mickenautsch S, Yengopal V, Banerjee A.** Atraumatic Restorative Treatment versus amalgam restoration longevity: a systematic review. Clinical Oral Investigations. 2009. Published online.
18. **Walkens CE Schuchard A.** Thermal and histologic response to high speed cutting in tooth structure. JADA, 1965; 71: 1451-1458.
19. **Lester KS.** Burs, teeth and hand instrument. Aust. Dent Journal 1978; 23(3): 231-236.
20. **Boston DW.** New device for selective dentin caries removal. Quintessence Int. 2003 Oct. 34(9): 678-85.

21. **Antunes LAA, Pedro RL Vieira ASB, Maia LC.** Effectiveness of high speed instrument and air abrasion on different dental substrates. Braz. Oral Res. 2008 Vol 22 no.3
22. **Schutzbank SG, Marchwinski M, Kronman JG, Goldman M, Clark RE.** In vitro study of the effect of GK-101 on the removal of carious materials. J Dent Res.1975; 54(4):907.
23. **Ericson D, Zimmerman M, Raber H, Gotrick B, Bornstien R, Thorell J.** Clinical evaluation of efficacy and safety of new method of chemomechanical removal of caries. A multicentre study. Caries res. 1999. May-June; 33(3):171-7.
24. **Maragakis GM, Hahn P, Hellwig E.** Clinical evaluation of chemomechanical caries removal in primary molars and its acceptance by patients. Caries Res. 2001; 35(3): 205-210.
25. **Burrow MF, Bokas J, Tanumihraja M, Tyas MJ.** Microtensile bond strength to caries – affected dentin treated with Carisolv. Aust Dent J 2008. Vol 48. Issue 2.p.110-114
26. **Sakoolnamarka R, Burrow MF, Kubo S, Tyas MJ.** Morphologic study of demineralised dentine after caries removal using two different methods. Aust Dent J. 2002 Jun; 47(2): 116-22.
27. **Rafique S, Fiske J, Banerjee A.** Clinical trial of an air abrasion chemo-mechanical operative procedure for restorative treatment of dental patients. Caries Res. 2003; 37(5): 360-364.
28. **Yazici AR, Atilla P, Ozgunaltay G, Muftuoglu S.** In vitro comparison of the efficacy of Carisolv and conventional rotary instrument in caries removal. J. Oral Rehabil. 2003; 30(12): 1177-1182.
29. **Azark B, Callaway A, Grundheber A, Stender E, Willershausen B.** Comparison of the efficacy of chemomechanical caries removal (Carisolv

TM) with that of conventional excavation in reducing the cariogenic flora. Int. J. Pediatric Dent. 2004; 14(3): 182-191.

30. **Fluckiger L, Waltimo T, Stich H, Lussi A.** Comparison of chemomechanical caries removal using Carisolv ™ or conventional hand excavation in deciduous teeth in vitro. Journal of Dentistry 2005, 33; 87-90.

31. **Balciuniene I, Sabalaite R, Juskiene I.** Chemomechanical caries removal for children. Stomatologija, Baltic Dental and Maxillofacial Journal 2005; 7: 40-4.

32. **Peters MC, Flamenbaum MH, Eboda NN, Feigal RJ, Inglehart MR.** Chemomechanical caries removal in children. Efficacy and efficacy. JADA 2006; 137(12): 1658-66.

33. **Chourio MAL, Zambrano O, Gonzalez H, Quero M.** Clinical randomized trial of chemomechanical caries removal (Carisolv ™). Int. J. Pediatric Dent. 2006; 16: 161-167.

34. **Pandit IK. Srivastava N, Gugnani N, Gupta M, Verma L.** Various methods of caries removal in children: A comparative clinical study. J. Indian Soc Pedod Prev Dent-Jun 2007.

35. **Inglehart MR, Habil P, Peters MC, Flamenbaum MH, Nnenna N, Eboda, Fiegal RJ.** Chemomechanical caries removal in children: an operator and pediatric patient's response. J Am Dent Assoc, Vol 138, No 1, 47-55.

36. **Subramanamiam P, Babu KLG, Neeraja G.** Comparison of the antimicrobial efficacy of chemomechanical caries removal (Carisolv ™) with that of conventional drilling in reducing cariogenic flora. J. Clin Pediatr Dent 2008. Vol 32, No. 3; p-215-219.

37. **Carrillo CM, Tanaka MH, Cesar MF, Camargo MAF, Juliano Y, Novo NF.** Use of papain gel in disabled patients. I. Dent. Child (Chic.) 2008 Sep-Dec; 75(3): 222-8.
38. **Bussadori SK, Guedes CC, Bruno MLH, Ramd.** Chemo-mechanical removal of caries in adolescent patient using a papain gel: Case report. J. Clin Pediatr Dent 2008. Vol 32, No. 3 p 177-180.
39. **Motta LJ, Martins MD, Porta KP, Bussadori SK.** Aesthetic restoration of deciduous anterior teeth after removal of carious tissue with Papacarie. Indian Journal of Dental research. 2009. Vol 20, Issue 1.p.117-120.
40. **Ricketts DNJ, Ekstrand KR, Kidd EAM, Larsen T.** Relating visual and radiographic ranked scoring systems for occlusal caries detection to histological and microbiologocal evidence. Operative Dentistry, 2002, 27 231-237.
41. **Hintze H, Wenzel A, Danielsen B, Nyvad B.** Reliability of visual examination, fibre-optic transillumination and bite wing radiography, and reproducibility of direct visual examination following tooth separation for the identification of cavitated carious lesions in contacting approximal surfaces. Caries Res 1998; 32: 204-209.
42. **Ericson D.** Efficacy of a new gel for chemo-mechanical caries removal. J Dent Res. 77:1252. Abstract 360, 1999.
43. **Nayak R, Sudha P.** Evaluation of three topical anaesthetic agents against pain: A clinical study. Indian J Dent Res 2006; 17:155-60.
44. AppendixApain/discomfortevaluationtool. www.amda.com/tools/library/whitepapers/.../appendix-a.pdf
45. **Malvin E Ring.** Dentistry an illustrated history. 2nd Edition, 1992; Harry N Abrams Inc. publishers.

46. **Strand M, Jokstad A.** Determinants of quality in operative dentistry. Crit Rev Biol Med. 1998; 9(4):464-79.
47. **Magalhes LS, Moreira AN.** Effectiveness and efficiency of chemomechanical carious dentine removal. Brazillian Dental Journal 2006,17 (1) 63-67.
48. **Habib CM, Kronman J, Goldman M.** A chemical evaluation of collagen and hydroxyproline alter treatment with GK-101 (N-chloroglycine). Pharmacol Ther Dent, v2,209-215.1975.
49. **Banerjee A, Watson TF, Kidd EAM.** Dentine caries excavation a review of current clinical technique. Br Dent J 2000; 188(9):476-482.
50. **Beeley JA, Yip HK, Stevenson AG.** Chemo-chemical caries removal a review of the techniques and latest developments. Br. Dent J 2000; 188(8):427-430.
51. **Banerjee A, Watson TF, Kidd EAM.** Dentin caries, Take it or leave it? Dental Update, 2000;27: 272-276.
52. **Candido LC.** Nova abordagem no tratamento de feridas. Sao Pualo: Senac-SP 2001. Available: http://www. Feridologo.com.br/curpapaina.htm [2003Dez].
53. **Mandelbaum SH, Santis EP, Mandelbaum MHS.** Cicatrization: current concepts and auxillary resources – Part II. An Bras Dermatol 2003; 78(5):525-542.
54. **Osato JA, Santiago LA, Remo GM, Caudra MS, Mori A.** Antimicrobial and antioxidant activities of unripe papaya. Life sci 1999; 53(17):1383-1389.
55. **Flindt M.** Health and safety aspects of working with enzymes. Process Biochem 1979; 13(8):3-7.

56. **Dawkins G, Hewitt H, Wint Y, Obiefuna PC, Wint B**. Antibacterial effects of carica papaya fruit on common wound organisms. West Indian Med J 2003; 52(4):290-292.
57. Chemomechanical caries removal: a comprehensive review of the literature. Int Dent J 2001; 5(4):291-29.
58. **Tonami K, Araki K, Mataki S, Kurosaki N**. Effects of chloramines and sodium hypochlorite on carious dentin. J Med Dent Sci 2003; 50(2).
59. **Silva LR, Tonolli G, Santos EM, Bussadori SK**. Avaliacao da biocompatibilidade in vitro de um novo biomaterial para remocao quimica e mecanica da carie. In: 20 Reuniao Anual SBPqO 2003.
60. **Pereira AS, Silva LR, Piccinini DPF, Santos EM, Bussadori SK**. Comparacao in vitro do potencial antimicrobiano de dois materiais para remocao quimico-mecanica da carie.
61. **Reda SH, Motta LFG, Bussadori SK**. Avaliacao do gel a base de papaina para remocao química e mecanica da lesao carie - Papacarie®.
62. **Health Care Products Manufacturer exporting direct from Brazil.** www.alibaba.com/product/health_care_products.html.
63. **Gordan Nikiforuk**. Epidemiology of Dental Caries. In: Understanding Dental caries, Etiology and Mechanism, Basic and Clinical Aspects. Karger Publications.
64. **Mariri BP, Levy SM, Warren JJ, Bergus GR, Broffitt B**. Medically administered, dietary habits, fluoride intake and dentals caries experience in primary dentition. Community Dent Epidemiol 2003;31:40-51.
65. **Mugonzibwa EA, Kuijpers JAM, Laine AMT**. Emergence of permanent teeth in Tanzanian children. Community Dent Oral Epidemol 2002; 30: 455-62.

66. **Mc Grath PA.** Review article- an assessment of children's pain. Pain 1987, 147-176.
67. Manual for the ART approach to control dental caries. Dental Health International. Nederland.
68. **Kakaboura A, Masouras C, Staikou O, Vougiouklakis G.** A comparative clinical study on the caries removal method. Quint. Int 2003; 34(4):269-271.
69. **Fure , Lingstrom P.** Evaluation of Carisolv for chemo mechanical removal of primary root caries in vivo. Caries Res. 2000; 34(3):275-280.
70. **Ziskind D, Kupietzky A, Beyth N.** First choice treatment alternatives for caries removal using the chemo-mechanical method. Quint. Int.2005; 36(1):9-14.
71. **Wewers ME, Lowe NK.** A critical review of visual analogue scales in the measurement of clinical phenomena. Research in Nursing and Health. V13(4).p227-236.
72. **Wade JB, Price DD, Hamer RM, Schwartz SM, Hart RP.** An emotional component analysis of chronic pain. Pain . 40.(1990), 303-310.
73. **Price DD, Harkins SW.** The combined use of Visual analogue scale and experimental pain in providing standardised assessment of clinical pain. Clin. J Pain. 3 (1987)3-11.
74. **Versloot J, Veerkal JS.** Dental discomfort questionnaire for going children before and after treatment. Acta Odontol Scand 2005; 63 (6), 367-76.
75. **Keele KD.** The pain chart. Lancet.1948 Jul 3;2(6514):6-8.
76. **Calvo AF, Rodrigues CR, Arana-Chaves VE.** Tempo gasto para remocao de carie em deciduous com metodos mecanico e quimico-mecanico e aspect da dentina em MEV. Resumen 074. Braz Oral Res 2005;19(suppl.):54.
77. **Torices SS, Gonzalez G, Queijo L, Ottati V, Martinez C, Freiria M.** Chemicalmechanical Caries removal using Papacarie restauration quality

evaluation. Preliminary report. The preliminary program for 2nd annual meeting of the IADR. Uruguayan Section, August 3, 2007.

78. **Splieth C, Rosin M, Gellissen B.** Determination of residual dentin caries after conventional and chemo mechanical caries removal with Carisolv. Clin. Oral Investing 2001; 5(4):250-253.

79. **Anusavice KJ, Kincheloe JE.** Comparison of pain associated with mechanical and chemo mechanical removal of caries. J Dent Res. 1987 Nov.66(11):1680-3.

80. **Guare RO.** Avaliacao de alteracoes comportamentais e fisiologicas durante a remocao de tecido cariado atraves dos metodos mecanico e quimico-mecanico (Carisolv TM) em criancas com syndrome de down. Sao Paulo. Faculdade de Odontologia de USP; 2004.Assessment of behavioural and physiological changes during caries removal by mechanical methods and chemicalmechanical (Carisolv TM) in children with down syndrome.

81. **Ayrton O.** Odontopediatria Fundamentos para la practica clinica. 2nd Sao Paulo:Premier. 1996. P67-70.

82. **Ferreira CM, Bonifacio KC, Froner IC, Ito IY.** Evaluation of the antimicrobial activity of three irrigating solutions in teeth with pulpal necrosis. Braz Dent J 1999; 10(1): 1-5.

83. **Miyagi SPH, Bussadori SK, Marques MM.** Reposta de fibroblastos pulpares humanos ao gel Papacarie ® "resumen PA69". RPG 2004,11(3):287.

84. **Barata TJE, Pereira LCG, Borges DLM, Lima AA, Navapro MFL.** Evaluation of Papacarie in ART restorations using Visual Analogue Scale. July 4 2008 Metro Toronto Convention.

85. **Lennon AM.** Fluorescence aided caries excavation (FACE) compared to conventional methods.Oper Dent 2003, 28: 341-345.

86. **Bergmann J, Leitao J, Kultje C, Bergmann D, Clode MJ.** Removing dentinal caries in deciduous teeth with Carisolv: a randomized, controlled prospective study with 6 months follow up comparing chemomechanical treatment with drilling. Oral Health Prev Dent 2005; 3(2) 105-11.
87. **Kavvadia K, Karagianni V, Polychronopoulou, Papagainnouli L.** Primary teeth caries removal using the Carisolv chemo-mechanical method. A clinical trial. Pediatric Dentistry, 2004,26(1):23-28.
88. **Allen KL, Lynch E, Petersson L, Borsboom.** Comparison of caries using Carisolv or a conventional slow speed rotary instrument. Caries Res. 1999; 33:313-315.
89. **Zinck JH, Mcinnes-Ledoux, Capdeboscq C, Weinberg R.** Chemo mechanical caries removal a clinical evaluation. Journal of Oral Rehabilitation, 1988;15:23-33.
90. **Yip HK, Beeley JA, Stevenson AG.** Mineral content of the dentine remaining after chemo mechanical caries removal. Caries Res 1995; 29(2) 111-7.
91. **Gurbuz T.** Pain related to mechanical and chemomechanical removal of caries in children. The Pain Clinic 2004;16(3).
92. **Singh KA, Moraes AB, Bovi AG.** Medo, anisiedade e controle relacionados ao tratamento odontologico. Pesq Odont Bras abr/jun 2000;14(2):131-6.

APPENDIX I

Visual Analogue Scale

0 —|—|—|—|—|—|—|—|—|— 100

APPENDIX- II

DEPARTMENT OF PEDODONTICS AND PREVENTIVE DENTISTRY
D.A.V. (C) DENTAL COLLEGE AND HOSPITAL,
YAMUNA NAGAR – 135001 [HARYANA]

Name of the patient……………………………………Age & Sex…………..……….

S/o, W/o, D/o………………………………………Address………………………..

Type of treatment……………….in Patient/Out Patient………………………….

Date………………………….

I acknowledge that my attending dentist has explained to me.

- The nature and benefits of proposed caries removal procedure.
- The consequence of not performing procedures.
- Significant complications of proposed procedures.
- Possible significant complications of proposed procedures.
- I have had the opportunity to ask questions to the dentist and all my questions have been answered to my satisfaction. Nobody has given me a promise or guarantee about results. I know it is my responsibility to openly discuss any problem with the dentist who gives me anesthesia.

Signature of Doctor   Signature of Patient   Date and Time

Parent/Guardian

The undersigned hereby consents to the above, on behalf of the patient, who is a minor or is unable to sign, because:

…………………………………. (Close Relative or Legal Guardian)

Name………………………..……….
Address……………………………….

Relation with the Patient………….

APPENDIX- III

COMPARATIVE CLINICAL EVALUATION OF VARIOUS CARIES REMOVING METHODS IN CHILDREN

NAME :

AGE/SEX :

OPD NO. :

DATE :

OCCUPATION :

ADDRESS :

TELEPHONE NO. :

DIAGNOSIS :

TREATMENT :

UNDER THE GUIDANCE OF :

CARIES REMOVAL METHOD USED:

- By hand instruments
- By bur
- By Carisolv
- By Papacarie

SCORES

1. EFFICACY

2. TIME TAKEN

3. VISUAL ANALOGUE SCALE

4. VERBAL PAIN SCALE

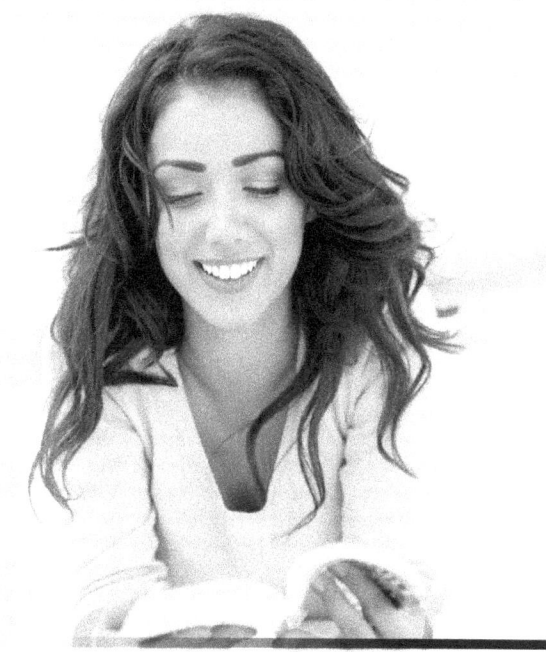

i want morebooks!

Buy your books fast and straightforward online - at one of world's fastest growing online book stores! Environmentally sound due to Print-on-Demand technologies.

Buy your books online at
www.get-morebooks.com

Kaufen Sie Ihre Bücher schnell und unkompliziert online – auf einer der am schnellsten wachsenden Buchhandelsplattformen weltweit! Dank Print-On-Demand umwelt- und ressourcenschonend produziert.

Bücher schneller online kaufen
www.morebooks.de

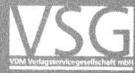

VDM Verlagsservicegesellschaft mbH
Heinrich-Böcking-Str. 6-8   Telefon: +49 681 3720 174   info@vdm-vsg.de
D - 66121 Saarbrücken   Telefax: +49 681 3720 1749   www.vdm-vsg.de

Lightning Source UK Ltd.
Milton Keynes UK
UKHW010638010421
381372UK00001B/136